ICF Core Sets

About the Authors

Jerome Bickenbach, PhD, LLB, is a steering committee member of the ICF Research Branch and was involved in the development of the ICF at the WHO and is a member of the Functioning and Disability Reference Group (FDRG) at WHO.

Alarcos Cieza, Psychologist, PhD, MPH, is a steering committee member of the ICF Research Branch. She has led the development process of several ICF Core Sets since 2001. She has also led the development of the ICF e-learning tool of WHO and participated in the development of other training materials and of the ICF Core Set-based documentation tools. She is a member of the Functioning and Disability Reference Group (FDRG) of WHO and has contributed to the ICF update and has led the measurement group.

Todd E. Davenport, PT, DPT, OCS, has applied the ICF and ICF Core Sets to physical therapy in the care of individuals with musculoskeletal health conditions.

Reuben Escorpizo, PT MSc, DPT, led the development of the ICF Core Set for Vocational Rehabilitation and has also collaborated on the validation of ICF Core Sets.

Monika Finger, PT MSc, participated in the development of the ICF Core Set for Vocational Rehabilitation and the development and validation of an ICF Core Set based questionnaire for vocational rehabilitation.

Andrea Glässel, PT BSc, MSc Neuroreha, MPH, participated in the development and validation of several ICF Core Sets. She provides ICF training in different health professional degree programs.

Miriam Lückenkemper, MA Psychology/Communication science, was involved in the development and validation of ICF-based measurements, manuals, and ICF Core Sets for Vocational Rehabilitation.

Pavel Ptyushkin, MD, MPH, worked for the ICF-focused Multidisciplinary Research Network on Health and Disability in Europe (MURINET) and participated in the development and validation of the ICF Core Sets for Traumatic Brain Injury and Bipolar Disorder. He has given ICF training workshops.

Alexandra Rauch, PT, Health scientist BSc, MPH, participated in the development and validation of several ICF Core Sets, ICF Core Set-based documentation tools and various ICF training materials. Leader of ICF training workshops.

Sean D. Rundell, PT MS, DPT, OCS, has applied the ICF Model and ICF Core Sets to physical therapy in the care of individuals with musculoskeletal health conditions.

Melissa Selb, (Vocational) Rehabilitation Counselor, MSc, is the Coordinator of the ICF Research Branch and has been a member of the organizational team of several ICF Core Set consensus conferences. She has given ICF training workshops.

Gerold Stucki, MD, MS, is Professor and Chair of the Department of Health Sciences and Health Policy at the University of Lucerne, Director of Swiss Paraplegic Research (SPF) and Director of the ICF Research Branch. As Co-Chair of the Functioning and Disability Reference Group (FDRG) of the WHO Family of International Classifications (WHO-FIC) Network and President of the International Society of Physical and Rehabilitation Medicine (ISPRM), he is promoting the implementation of the ICF in medicine, rehabilitation, and the health sector at large. Towards this goal he initiated the ICF Core Set project and has guided their development as a member of the steering committee.

ICF Core Sets

Manual for Clinical Practice

Editors

Jerome Bickenbach

Alarcos Cieza

Alexandra Rauch

Gerold Stucki

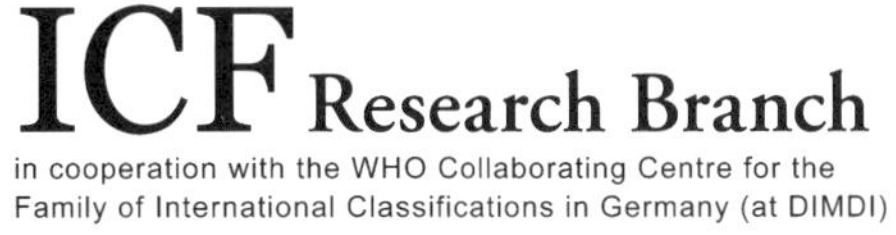

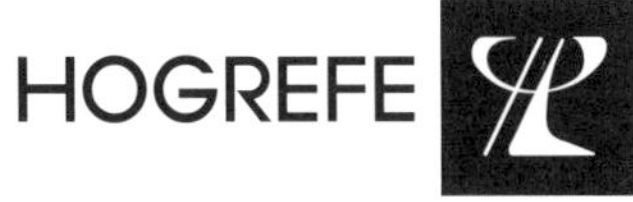

Library of Congress Cataloging-in-Publication Data

is available via the Library of Congress Marc Database under the
Library of Congress Control Number 2012935835

Library and Archives Canada Cataloguing in Publication

ICF core sets : manual for clinical practice / editors,
Jerome Bickenbach ... [et al.].

"ICF Research Branch in cooperation with the WHO
Collaborating Centre for the Family of International
Classifications in Germany (at DIMDI)."
Includes bibliographical references and index.
ISBN 978-0-88937-431-7

1. Human physiology--Classification--Handbooks,
manuals, etc. 2. Human anatomy--Classification--Handbooks,
manuals, etc. 3. Disability evaluation--Classification--
Handbooks, manuals, etc. I. Bickenbach, Jerome Edmund

R123.I34 2012 612.001'2 C2012-902000-1

PUBLISHING OFFICES
USA: Hogrefe Publishing, 875 Massachusetts Avenue, 7th Floor, Cambridge, MA 02139
Phone (866) 823-4726, Fax (617) 354-6875; E-mail customerservice@hogrefe-publishing.com
EUROPE: Hogrefe Publishing, Merkelstr. 3, 37085 Göttingen, Germany
Phone +49 551 99950-0, Fax +49 551 99950-425, E-mail publishing@hogrefe.com

SALES & DISTRIBUTION
USA: Hogrefe Publishing, Customer Services Department,
30 Amberwood Parkway, Ashland, OH 44805
Phone (800) 228-3749, Fax (419) 281-6883, E-mail customerservice@hogrefe.com
EUROPE: Hogrefe Publishing, Merkelstr. 3, 37085 Göttingen, Germany
Phone +49 551 99950-0, Fax +49 551 99950-425, E-mail publishing@hogrefe.com

OTHER OFFICES
CANADA: Hogrefe Publishing, 660 Eglinton Ave. East, Suite 119-514, Toronto, Ontario, M4G 2K2
SWITZERLAND: Hogrefe Publishing, Länggass-Strasse 76, CH-3000 Bern 9

Hogrefe Publishing
Incorporated and registered in the Commonwealth of Massachusetts, USA, and in Göttingen, Lower Saxony, Germany

Printed and bound in Germany

ISBN 978-0-88937-431-7

Table of Contents

The documentation form to create a functioning profile mentioned in this manual is also available in an open access interactive web-based format www.icf-core-sets.org

Preface

Gerold Stucki

The diagnosis of health conditions and the assessment of an individual's functioning are at the core of clinical practice. For the diagnosis and classification of health conditions, health professionals have relied for more than 100 years on the World Health Organization's (WHO) *International Classification of Diseases* (ICD), whose 11th edition is currently under way. For the assessment and description of functioning, health professionals have been able to turn to the ICD's companion volume, the *International Classification of Functioning, Disability and Health* (ICF) for the past 10 years. The ICD and the ICF are currently used for health statistics so that mortality, morbidity and disability data can be collected in a uniform and internationally comparable fashion. There are a variety of other uses for these classifications, such as programme eligibility and reimbursement. Most importantly, however, the ICF has great potential for enhancing clinical practice by providing a standardized description of functioning by means of ICF-based tools, such as those described here. This information is central for all features of clinical practice: these data structure the clinical assessment of functioning, the assignment to health services and health interventions and the management of services and interventions, including outcome evaluation. In this manual we focus on the description of functioning for which standardization is of crucial importance, both for consistent practice and for comparable health outcomes.

When the ICF was endorsed by the World Health Assembly in 2001, it represented the outcome of a unique international collaborative exercise that produced not only a paradigm shift in our understanding of functioning and disability, but also a complete classificatory tool that, for the first time, made health and disability information comparable around the globe. Yet, by constructing an exhaustive classification, it was clear that the ICF was not directly usable as a practical tool since, in daily practice, clinicians need only a fraction of the categories found in the ICF. Responding to the need for practical ICF-based tools for clinical practice, the ICF Core Set project was begun soon after in 2001.[1–2]

The ICF Core Sets provide health professionals with invaluable tools tailored for specific health care areas. In this manual, health professionals will find practical guidance on how to apply ICF Core Sets in their clinical practice in order to structure the clinical description and assessment of functioning. Although ICF Core Sets are intended for all health practitioners, the emphasis in this manual is on the needs of health professionals who apply the ICF Core Sets in the context of rehabilitation. The manual is inherently multi-professional and may be used not only by practitioners working in different settings but also by students in the health professions, their teachers and their mentors.

To facilitate the use of the manual, each chapter can be read on its own. The manual starts with an introduction to the concept of functioning as the lived experience of health. It then provides an introduction to the ICF and the process and scope of the development of the ICF Core Sets. A theoretical chapter outlining the principals that govern the use of the ICF Core Sets in practice is followed by a series of use cases illustrating how to apply the ICF Core Sets in different contexts. To facilitate the use of the ICF Core Sets in clinical practice, the manual also includes a CD containing over 1,400 pages of documentation forms.

The editors and authors of this manual are enthusiastic about the enormous potential that the implementation of the ICF and the ICF Core Sets has to better understand patients' problems and how to best address their needs. We recognize that this manual would not have been possible without the outstanding effort of health professionals around the world and the excellent support provided by the Classification, Terminology and Standards Team at WHO, led by Dr. Bedirhan Üstün and coordinated by Nenad Kostanjsek. We wish to commend everyone who has contributed to this outstanding and valuable practical tool.

The ICF and the ICF Core Sets are still new and their use in clinical practice is still challenging. We would therefore like to encourage users of this manual to become involved in the further development of the ICF and the ICF Core Sets by collaborating with the ICF Research Branch in cooperation with the WHO Collaboration Centre for the Family of International Classifications in Germany (at DIMDI), www.icf-research-branch.org. Let's learn from each other!

1 What Is Functioning and Why Is It Important

Jerome Bickenbach

Everyone knows what health is, although we are all a bit vague about it. A researcher who had spent years defining health gave up saying that "it seems to be impossible to devise a concept of health which is rich enough to be nutritious and yet not so rich as to be indigestible".[3] Although the World Health Organization's definition of health as "a state of complete physical, mental and social well-being and not merely the absence of disease or infirmity" is famous, when it comes to collecting information about people's health, assessing patients, planning health interventions and describing the outcomes we want, no one actually uses this definition. To be practical about health information, we need a more concrete notion of "health". We need to focus on what matters about one's health. Longevity certainly matters, but for most of us, our health is more about what we can do or not do in our lives. Health, in short, is about how we function in our day to day lives. In order to denote this positive and practical aspect of health, WHO used the term "functioning", which is the foundation for the *International Classification of Functioning, Disability and Health* (ICF).

What does the WHO mean by functioning? Firstly, the WHO notion is both narrower and broader than the ordinary English term "functioning". It is narrower because it only applies to humans, but far broader because it captures all body functions and body structures and everything that people do (actions, tasks, skills) as well as all the things they are or aspire to be (parents, workers, voters). In the following chapters, the specific details of how the WHO concept of functioning operates in the ICF will be carefully set out, since these details are crucial for understanding the ICF Core Sets and their application. Here we look only at how WHO intends the concept of functioning to be used.

For the WHO, functioning is a set of specific domains of human functioning – once again, body functions and body structures and the things people do and the things people are or aspire to be. These domains of functioning are the categories that are the items in the ICF classification. Secondly, the WHO understands functioning to be a continuous concept, that is, a concept of "more or less", measurable along a continuum from complete (or total) functioning to complete absence of (or no) functioning. In other words, when people experience difficulties in functioning the result is disability, in the WHO sense of that word. The word "disability" has suffered the plight of being defined in countless different ways, by people concerned about theory as well as people concerned about practice. Even within the health professions, there is really no consensus about what disability means. It was for that reason that the WHO outlined its notion of disability defining disability in terms of functioning; in particular, as that level of functioning that is below a determined threshold along a continuum, for each domain, between completely present and completely absent.

Where that threshold is placed is not the WHO's decision, but is a matter for science and practice, epidemiology and population-based norms. It is also, it must be said, an economic and political judgment. It is clear, though, that where the threshold for disability lies is not the WHO's decision but has been left to each country to determine and justify to the community of health professionals and practitioners. Obviously, the complete absence of functioning is disability, so drawing no threshold at all would be impossible to justify. Putting the threshold close to complete functioning, would also be impossible to justify. So, the threshold is somewhere in the middle of the continuum, most likely closer to the "complete" absence end. Figure 1 is a graphical depiction, along a continuum, of the relationship between the WHO's conception of functioning and disability.

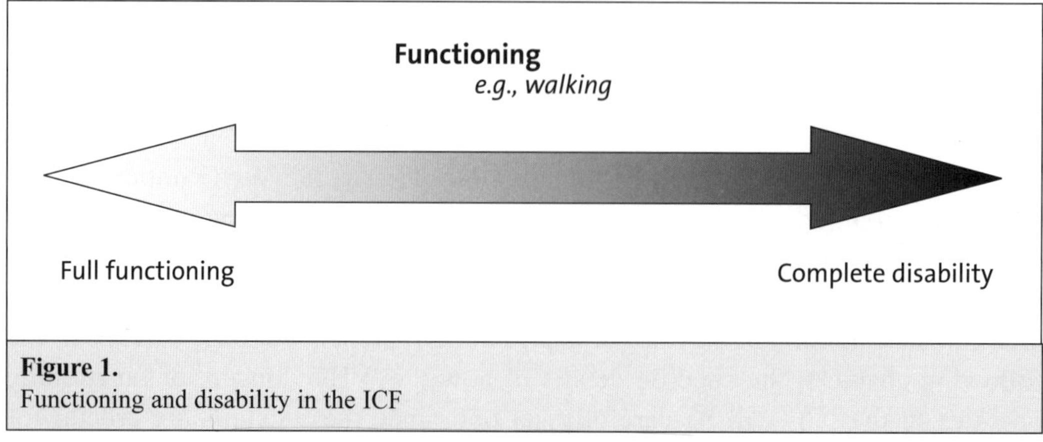

Figure 1.
Functioning and disability in the ICF

Why should the notion of functioning matter to health professionals? First and foremost, functioning is what matters to the health professionals' patients. Patients are not so much concerned to know medical facts; they want to know if they will be able to walk or see their friends across the street or get a job. All of us think of health as important because of how our health affects everything that we do in our lives. Secondly, there is no better description of outcomes of health interventions than improvements in functioning. Finally, we know that problems in functioning can predict both the objective need for health services and the subjective desire for these services. Administratively, therefore, health-system planning depends on good information about functioning.

In actual clinical and public health, uses of the WHO notion of functioning meet the challenges of descriptive data collection and analysis. At both the individual and the population levels, functioning describes the outcome of the four main public health strategies: prevention, cure, rehabilitation and support. We seek to improve functioning, either as a primary outcome (cure and rehabilitation) or as a related outcome (prevention and support).[4] Functioning is also valuable for the clinical assessment of individuals. As we shall show in the following chapters, the ICF functioning framework offers a common terminology and conceptual model for the improvement of clinical and patient-oriented assessment instruments. Thus, for example, the international network OMERACT (Outcome Measures in Rheumatology) has adopted the ICF as the reference model to understand what to measure when thinking about the lived experience of rheumatoid arthritis.[5] The ICF is also the basis for the ICF Core Sets for which this manual provides guidance for use in practice.

2 Introduction to the International Classification of Functioning, Disability and Health

Alexandra Rauch, Miriam Lückenkemper and Alarcos Cieza

In May 2001, the *International Classification of Functioning, Disability and Health* (ICF)[6] of the WHO was endorsed by the World Health Assembly. The ICF provides a comprehensive and standardized framework and language for the description of *functioning* and *disability*. As introduced in Chapter 1, functioning is the lived experience of health. To better understand functioning, the ICF offers a multidimensional approach based on the interaction of components of the person and the person's environment. As a classification, the ICF systematically classifies and groups components of functioning and environmental factors, each of which is composed of domains (chapters and blocks) and categories. Qualifiers are provided to describe the extent of the problems in functioning, that is, the extent of disability denoted in each domain and category. This chapter provides an introduction to the basic concepts of the ICF.

2.1. The Integrative Model of Functioning, Disability and Health

Functioning is the umbrella term for Body Functions, Body Structures and Activities and Participation. Disability refers to impairments in Body Functions and Body Structures, limitations in Activities and restrictions in Participation (the definitions of all these components are presented in Table 1). Most importantly, although functioning is associated with a health condition (which includes diseases, disorders and injuries), it is not conceptualized as the direct consequence of a health condition but rather the result of the interaction between a health condition and contextual factors (Environmental and Personal Factors). The interaction among these components is dynamic and bidirectional; changes in one component may influence one or more of the other components. This understanding is depicted by the integrative biopsychosocial model of the ICF in Figure 2.

The ICF model, as depicted in Figure 2, illustrates the essential role of Environmental and Personal Factors for a person's level of functioning and disability. Environmental Factors can act as *barriers* (producing or increasing the severity of a disability) or as *facilitators* (improving or even eliminating a disability). For this reason, Environmental Factors must always be taken into account when describing a person's level of functioning.

With this model, the ICF contributes to a better understanding of functioning and disability and so offers a better approach to describing the lived experience of health. This model also serves as the basis for the classification of functioning.

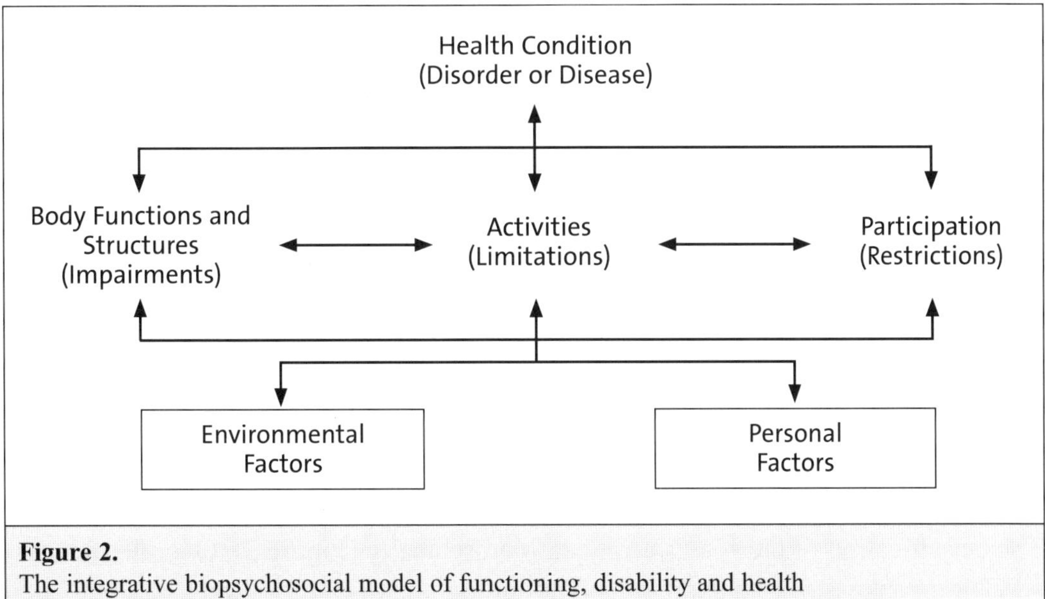

Figure 2.
The integrative biopsychosocial model of functioning, disability and health

Table 1.
Definitions of the components of the model of functioning and disability

Positive	Negative
Body Functions are the physiological functions of body systems (including psychological functions) **Body Structures** are anatomical parts of the body such as organs, limbs and their components	**Impairments** are problems in body functions or structures such as significant deviation or loss
Activity is the execution of a task or action by an individual	**Activity limitations** are difficulties an individual may have in executing activities
Participation is involvement in a life situation	**Participation restrictions** are problems an individual may experience in involvement in life situations
Facilitators	**Barriers**
Environmental Factors make up the physical, social and attitudinal environment in which people live and conduct their lives and can act as facilitators or barriers	
Personal Factors are the particular background of an individual's life and living and comprise features of the individual that are not part of a health condition or health state	

Like all standard classifications in the WHO's *Family of International Classifications* (WHOFIC)[7], the ICF provides a standard language for the description of functioning by classifying all relevant components of functioning and the environmental factors. Health conditions (disorders or diseases) are a component of the integrative model of functioning, disability and health and can be classified using the *International Classification of Diseases* (ICD).[8] Since the ICD and the ICF are thus complementary, users are advised to use them together to describe both the health condition and its impact on a person's functioning.

2.2. The Structure and Codes of the ICF Classification

The classification of the ICF is arranged hierarchically (Figure 3). Overall, the classification consists of two parts: (1) "functioning and disability" and (2) "contextual

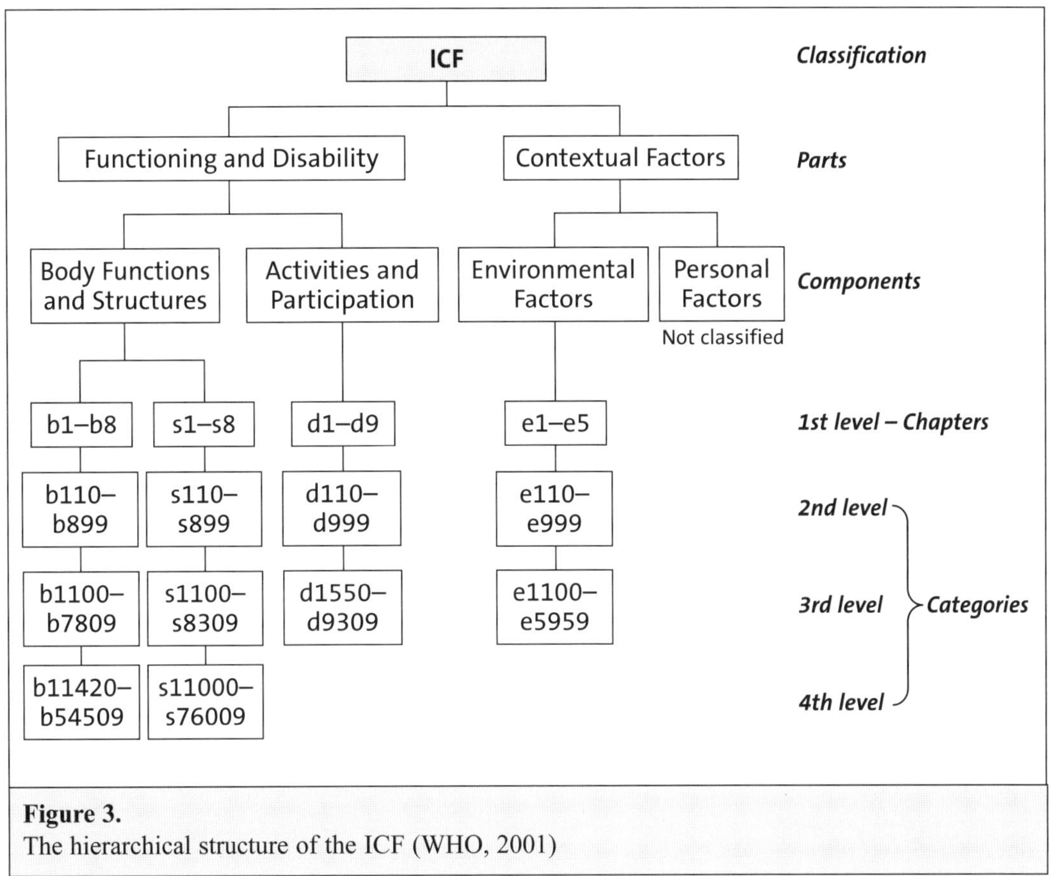

Figure 3.
The hierarchical structure of the ICF (WHO, 2001)

factors", each with two *components*: Part 1 consists of "Body Functions and Body Structures" and "Activities and Participation", and Part 2 consists of "Environmental Factors" and "Personal Factors". Although Personal Factors are included in the integrative model of functioning, disability and health, they are not as yet classified in the ICF.

In all of the classified components, *chapters* represent the 1st level of the classification. For coding, each chapter is subdivided into the basic elements of the classification, called *categories*, which are organized in hierarchically arranged 2nd, 3rd and 4th levels.

The codes of chapters and categories constitute the common classificatory language that can be applied unequivocally across countries, languages, cultures and professions for data collection and comparison. ICF codes are composed of a prefix (**b** for Body Functions, **s** for Body Structure, **d** for Activity and Participation and **e** for Environmental Factors) followed by a numeric code that consists of one digit for the 1st or chapter level, three digits for the 2nd, four for the 3rd and five for the 4th level, as in the example below.

b2 Sensory functions and pain	1st level chapter
b280 Sensation of pain	2nd level category
b2801 Pain in body part	3rd level category
b28010 Pain in head and neck **b28011** Pain in chest **b28012** Pain in stomach or abdomen **b28013** Pain in back **b28014** Pain in upper limb **b28015** Pain in lower limb **b28016** Pain in joints	4th level categories

The hierarchical organization of the classification allows users to choose either a broader description (e.g. by using a 1st level chapter or a 2nd level category) or a more detailed description (e.g. by using a 3rd or 4th level category) of an area of functioning. The level of specificity increases with each lower level as the example above shows. The hierarchical organization allows users to choose the level of specificity required for their needs.

For all categories, except those in Body Structures, definitions and inclusions and exclusions are provided as shown in the following example:

d510 Washing oneself

Washing and drying one's whole body or body parts, using water and appropriate cleaning and drying materials or methods, such as bathing, showering, washing hands and feet, face and hair, and drying with a towel.

Inclusions: washing body parts, the whole body; and drying oneself

Exclusions: caring for body parts (d520); toileting (d530)

The definitions and inclusions provide a detailed description of the meaning of the category and help practitioners use the ICF. The exclusions help to differentiate between related ICF categories.

To provide a convenient structure to the classification, chapters are often subdivided into *blocks* of categories. Blocks organize categories into common themes, as for example the block *Muscle functions (b730–b749)* comprising *b730 Muscle power functions*, *b735 Muscle tone functions*, *b740 Muscle endurance functions* and *b749 Muscle functions, other specified and unspecified*; or the block Household tasks (d630–d649) comprising *d630 Preparing meals*, *d640 Doing housework* and *d649 Household tasks, other specified and unspecified*. Blocks are not part of the structure of the classification and usually are not used for coding purposes.

While the categories of functioning classified in the ICF provide health and health-related domains it is essential to use the ICF qualifiers to capture all of the information for describing the extent of problems in functioning or disability. Although Personal Factors are not classified, users may assess and describe them in a manner that is suitable for their use.

2.3. ICF Qualifiers

In all the components of functioning (Body Functions, Body Structures, Activities and Participation), the first qualifier describes the extent of a problem in functioning – more precisely, it denotes the range from full functioning (no problem) to complete disability (complete problem), including the intermediate levels of mild, moderate and severe disability. “No problem” in functioning is used to denote the absence of a problem, understood to include optimal, full or even outstanding functioning. In the Environmental Factors, the first qualifier denotes the amount of positive (facilitator) or negative (barrier) impact of the Environmental Factor on functioning. An Environmental Factor is rated as a barrier because of its negative impact on functioning (e.g. the impact of bad air quality on respiration) or its absence (e.g. the impact of lack of support on performing housework). In some situations, the description of functioning or levels of disability or the impact of the environment is not possible due to a lack of information or the inapplicability of an ICF category. In these situations, the codes **.8** and **.9** are used. For all components, the description of functioning or levels of disability uses the following *generic scale* (Table 2).

To be meaningful, an ICF code requires at least one qualifier. Hence, an ICF code (composed of the letter and numeric code) is completed by at least the first qualifier placed after a dot following the numeric code, e.g. b28016**.3** (severe impairment in pain in joints). In the case of an environmental facilitator, the dot alone denotes a barrier and the plus (+) sign denotes a facilitator, e.g. e310+**4** (complete facilitator in the area of immediate family).

Other qualifiers are available for all components, except Body Functions (Table 3). Body Structures may be qualified with three qualifiers (first qualifier = extent of impairment, second qualifier = nature of impairment, third qualifier = location of impairment). For example, the ICF code **s7501.412** describes a complete impairment (**4**) due to total absence (**1**) of the left (**2**) lower leg (s7501).

For Activities and Participation, two qualifiers are required. The first qualifier records the level of performance of the area of Activities and Participation and the second the person’s capacity. Performance describes what an individual actually does in his or her current environment in light of the positive or negative impact of

Table 2.
Generic scale of the ICF qualifiers

First Qualifiers for Body Functions, Body Structures, and Activities and Participation:		
xxx.**0** NO problem	(none, absent, negligible,...)	0–4%
xxx.**1** MILD problem	(slight, low,...)	5–24%
xxx.**2** MODERATE problem	(medium, fair,...)	25–49%
xxx.**3** SEVERE problem	(high, extreme,...)	50–95%
xxx.**4** COMPLETE problem	(total,...)	96–100%
xxx.**8** not specified (used when there is insufficient information for the description of the extent of the problem)		
xxx.**9** not applicable (used when the category is applicable, e.g. in ‘b650 Menstruation functions’ for men)		
Qualifiers for Environmental Factors:		
xxx.**0** NO barrier	xxx+**0** NO facilitator	
xxx.**1** MILD barrier	xxx+**1** MILD facilitator	
xxx.**2** MODERATE barrier	xxx+**2** MODERATE facilitator	
xxx.**3** SEVERE barrier	xxx+**3** SUBSTANTIAL facilitator	
xxx.**4** COMPLETE barrier	xxx+**4** COMPLETE facilitator	
xxx.**8** barrier, not specified	xxx+**8** facilitator, not specified	
xxx.**9** not applicable	xxx.**9** not applicable	

Environmental Factors (including all aspects of the physical, social and attitudinal world). Capacity, by contrast, describes an individual’s inherent or intrinsic ability to perform a task or an action. To describe a person’s true capacity, the second qualifier describes capacity, the intrinsic ability of the person, without assistive devices, personal assistance or any other Environmental Factor acting as a facilitator or barrier. A neutralized environment, e.g. a test setting, is arguably the best suitable environment to obtain information about capacity. The difference between performance and capacity reflects the impact of Environmental Factors on functioning in the individual’s environment. For example, the ICF code d450.**13** describes a person’s capacity to walk as severely limited (**3** = severe problem in capacity) but the **1** (= mild problem with performance) indicates that the limitation in capacity is compensated by some Environmental Factor, for example a walking assistive device. More detailed information can be added with two optional qualifiers: a third qualifier to describe capacity with assistance and a fourth qualifier to describe performance without assistance.

Environmental Factors are quantified by only one qualifier. The impact on functioning or levels of disability can be positive when the factor is a facilitator or

Table 3.
Overview of qualifiers for the components of functioning and Environmental Factors

Component	1st Qualifier	2nd Qualifier	3rd Qualifier
Body Functions	**Extent of impairment** 0 = NO impairment 1 = MILD impairment 2 = MODERATE impairment 3 = SEVERE impairment 4 = COMPLETE impairment 8 = not specified 9 = not applicable	–	–
Body Structures	**Extent of impairment** 0 = NO impairment 1 = MILD impairment 2 = MODERATE impairment 3 = SEVERE impairment 4 = COMPLETE impairment 8 = not specified 9 = not applicable	**Nature of impairment** 0 = no change in structure 1 = total absence 2 = partial absence 3 = additional part 4 = aberrant dimension 5 = discontinuity 6 = deviating position 7 = qualitative changes in structure, including accumulation of fluid 8 = not specified 9 = not applicable	**Location of impairment** 0 = more than one region 1 = right 2 = left 3 = both sides 4 = front 5 = back 6 = proximal 7 = distal 8 = not specified 9 = not applicable
Activities and Participation	**Extent of difficulty in performance** 0 = NO difficulty 1 = MILD difficulty 2 = MODERATE difficulty 3 = SEVERE difficulty 4 = COMPLETE difficulty 8 = not specified 9 = not applicable	**Extent of difficulty in capacity** 0 = NO difficulty 1 = MILD difficulty 2 = MODERATE difficulty 3 = SEVERE difficulty 4 = COMPLETE difficulty 8 = not specified 9 = not applicable	

Table 3. Continued

Component	1st Qualifier	2nd Qualifier	3rd Qualifier
Environmental Factors	**Extent of the impact of the environment** 0 = NO barrier 1 = MILD barrier 2 = MODERATE barrier 3 = SEVERE barrier 4 = COMPLETE barrier 8 = barrier, not specified 9 = not applicable or +0 = NO facilitator +1 = MILD facilitator +2 = MODERATE facilitator +3 = SUBSTANTIAL facilitator +4 = COMPLETE facilitator +8 = facilitator, not specified 9 = not applicable	–	–

negative when it is a barrier. To denote this difference, a facilitator is marked with a plus sign instead of the dot (+X) and a barrier follows the dot (.X), hence e310+**2** means moderate facilitator "Immediate family" and e310.**2** means moderate barrier "Immediate family".

Qualifiers complete an ICF code and provide the full description of a person's functioning or level of disability. If standardized instruments or other sources of information are used to assess the level of functioning in a category, the results of the measure can be "translated" into a qualifier. Thus, using qualifiers facilitates a common understanding of the description of a person's level of functioning. Furthermore, the use of qualifiers makes it possible to develop functioning profiles as illustrated by the use cases in Chapter 5.

The ICF is an international classification standard and scientific tool for the description of functioning and disability. The application of the ICF contributes to the standardization of data and facilitates data collection and comparison. Since the ICF is a complete and exhaustive classification, however, it may be impractical when used in daily clinical practice. To address this problem, practical tools are required that are "tailored to the needs of the users without forgoing the information needed for health statistics and health reporting".[9] The ICF Core Sets have been developed to meet this need.

Summary Box

- The integrative *biopsychosocial model of functioning, disability and health* is the basis of the ICF.
- The model describes *dynamic interactions* between the components Body Functions, Body Structures, Activities and Participation, and Environmental and Personal Factors.
- Functioning is the result of the *interaction between a health condition and contextual factors* (Environmental and Personal Factors).
- The ICF is divided in two parts: (1) functioning and disability and (2) contextual factors each comprising *two components*: Part 1 = Body Functions and Body Structures and Activities and Participation, Part 2 = Environmental and Personal Factors.
- There are *four levels in the classification*: the 1st level is represented by chapters which are further subdivided in 2nd, 3rd and 4th level categories.
- *ICF qualifiers* describe the range from full functioning ("no problem") to extent of a problem (levels of disability) ranging from "mild", "moderate" or "severe problem" to "complete problem".
- An ICF code requires at least one qualifier to provide meaningful information.
- Activities and Participation are typically rated with two qualifiers, the first describing *performance* and the second describing *capacity*.
- For Environmental Factors, the qualifier rates the extent that factors act as *facilitators* or *barriers* to functioning.

3 ICF Core Sets

Pavel Ptyushkin, Melissa Selb and Alarcos Cieza

A classification needs to be exhaustive by its very nature. As a standard classification, the ICF is exhaustive in its coverage of the complete spectrum of health and health-related domains that make up the experience of functioning. With more than 1,400 categories, the ICF fulfils the formal criteria of exhaustiveness, especially in relation to the scope of covered domains. However, with exhaustiveness often comes complexity and impracticability. A common criticism of the ICF is that it is too comprehensive and too complicated for use in daily practice.

This obvious requirement of practicability was the primary motivation for the WHO to work in partnership with the ICF Research Branch in cooperation with the WHO Collaborating Centre for the Family of International Classifications in Germany (at the German Institute of Medical Documentation and Information or DIMDI) to develop ICF Core Sets.[10] An ICF Core Set is a selection of categories from the full ICF classification that provides a user-friendly tool for describing functioning and disability that has been developed by means of a scientifically-structured process. ICF Core Sets have been developed for various health care contexts (acute, post-acute and long-term) and for various health conditions and condition groups.[11] In most cases, they include ICF categories of the 2nd and 3rd level, but sometimes this level of precision was too precise so chapters are used (e.g. *d5 Self-care* in the Brief ICF Core Set for Traumatic Brain Injury). Sometimes it was felt useful to use chapter blocks (e.g. *d810–d839 Education* in the Brief and Comprehensive ICF Core Set for Inflammatory Bowel Diseases). By contrast, some ICF Core Sets include detailed categories up to the 4th level (e.g. *b28016 Pain in joints* in the Brief and Comprehensive ICF Core Set for Rheumatoid Arthritis).

Although the ICF Core Sets were developed to be used in any context in which a description of functioning and disability is necessary, in this manual we focus on their use in clinical practice. Most clinicians are familiar with and use the *International Classification of Diseases* (ICD) for describing health conditions diagnostically.[8] But the ICF is also increasingly being used in clinical practice. The joint use of ICD and ICF takes advantage of the beneficial synergy between the two classifications. Using both ensures that both diagnostic information and information about the lived experience of health are included to optimize our understanding of the true impact of a health condition.[12]

In clinical practice, the purpose of an ICF Core Set is to make the ICF practical for everyday use by presenting the most relevant ICF categories for a particular health condition, condition group and healthcare context. Use of the ICF Core Sets in clinical practice supports the interdisciplinary and comprehensive description of functioning by helping professionals caring for a patient to consider every potentially relevant aspect of functioning at every stage of an assessment, even in areas of functioning beyond their discipline.[13]

3.1. ICF Core Sets Development Process

The ICF Core Sets were developed by means of a rigorous, multi-method scientific process, represented by the steps shown in Figure 4.

Evidence was first gathered by means of four preparatory studies – an empirical multicenter study, a systematic literature review, a qualitative study and an expert survey. The *empirical multicenter study* identified the most common problems experienced by the target group of individuals by applying the ICF checklist. The *systematic literature review* summarized the international scientific literature on the particular health condition, health condition group or healthcare context. The *expert survey* identified problems of targeted individuals considered relevant by the experts

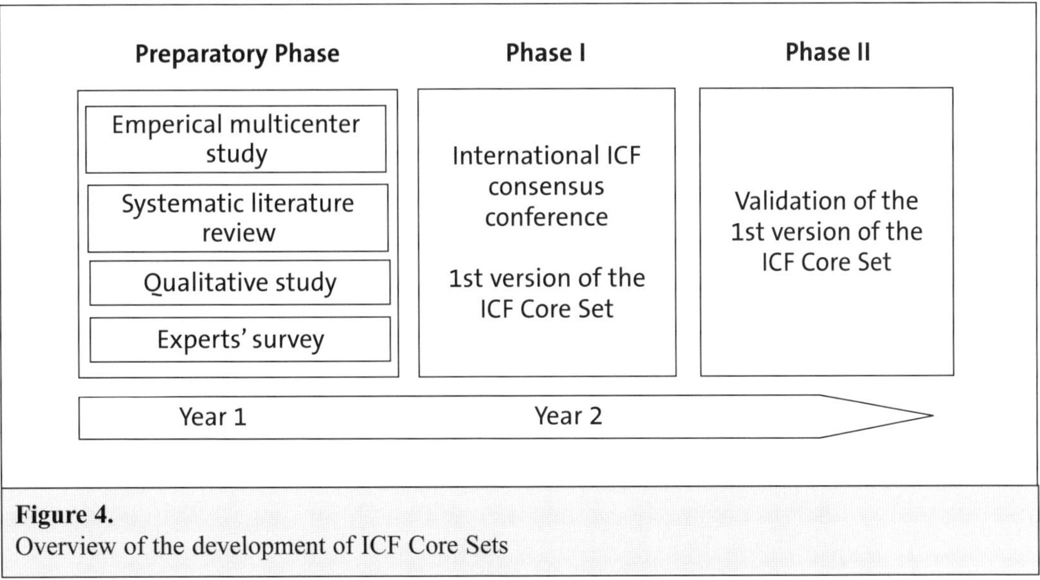

Figure 4.
Overview of the development of ICF Core Sets

and professionals who treat them. While these studies addressed the perspective of professionals and researchers, the *qualitative study* reflected the view of persons living with the health conditions. The results of the preparatory studies served as the starting point for a structured decision-making and consensus process at an international conference, during which participating health professionals and other experts decided on which ICF categories were to be included in the first version of the ICF Core Set.[14–25] The validation of ICF Core Sets is an ongoing process that incorporates the perspectives of different health professionals and relies on a variety of statistical approaches as well as patient-oriented, focused studies. This process is at different stages for the existing ICF Core Sets.

It is important to remember that an ICF Core Set offers a list of the most relevant ICF categories to assess patients with specific health conditions or in a specific healthcare context, it does not prevent the user from adding additional ICF categories if these are thought necessary for the user's purposes. Also, importantly, an ICF Core Set does not address the question of "how to measure" the ICF categories contained in it, but only "what to measure". It is noteworthy, therefore, to appreciate what an ICF Core Set is and what it is not, which is summarized in Table 4.

Table 4.
Overview of what ICF Core Sets are and are not

An ICF Core Set...	
does not replace the use of the whole ICF...	...but provides an approach that facilitates the practical use of the ICF.
does not go back to a causal model of the consequences of disease...	...but addresses functioning in light of a health condition.
has not been developed to be used exclusively in clinical practice...	...but in any context in which a description of functioning is necessary.
advises users which aspects of functioning to describe in patients with selected health conditions or in specific context...	...but does not tell users how to measure these aspects of functioning.

3.2. Available ICF Core Sets

The majority of ICF Core Sets have been developed to describe the functioning and disability of persons who experience a health condition (e.g. multiple sclerosis, depression) in specific healthcare contexts (acute, post-acute and long-term).

To date, thirty-one ICF Core Sets have been developed.[26] They are presented in Table 5 below. (The ICF Core Set development projects are still ongoing for hearing loss and lower limb amputation.)

Table 5.
Currently available ICF Core Sets

Acute Care	Post-Acute Care	Long-Term Care
Neurological conditions[27]	Neurological conditions[28–29]	Multiple sclerosis[30] Stroke (also as a cardiopulmonary condition)[31] Traumatic brain injury[32]
	Spinal cord injury[33]	Spinal cord injury[34]
Cardiopul-monary conditions[35]	Cardiopulmonary conditions[36]	Chronic ischemic heart disease[37] Diabetes mellitus[38] Obesity[39] Obstructive pulmonary diseases[40]
Musculoskeletal conditions[41]	Musculoskeletal conditions[42]	Ankylosing spondylitis[43] Chronic widespread pain[44] Low back pain[45] Osteoarthritis[46] Osteoporosis[47] Rheumatoid arthritis[48]
Acute inflamma-tory arthritis[49]		
	For geriatric patients[50]	
		Bipolar disorders[51]
		Depression[52]
		Breast cancer[53]
		Head and neck cancer[54]
		Hand conditions[55]
		Inflammatory bowel diseases[56]
		Sleep[57]
	Vocational rehabilitation[58]	

3.2.1. ICF Core Sets for the Acute Healthcare Context

The acute healthcare context is *the period of time immediately following an injury or onset of a health condition* and preceding the early post-acute context. The *ICF*

Core Sets for the acute healthcare context – for neurological, cardiopulmonary and musculoskeletal conditions, and for acute inflammatory arthritis – are intended for use by physicians, nurses, therapists and other health professionals involved in acute care, including those specialized in rehabilitation care provision.[28, 59] The duration of stay in an acute healthcare setting is usually short and focused on solving the most urgent functioning problems. ICF Core Sets for the acute care setting guide clinicians through this problem-solving process, ensuring that no crucial aspect of functioning is overlooked. ICF Core Sets in the acute healthcare context can also help to identify necessary follow-up treatment.

3.2.2. ICF Core Sets for the Post-Acute Healthcare Context

The post-acute healthcare context refers to any kind of healthcare setting (e.g. acute hospital, rehabilitation centre, ambulatory care) in which initial comprehensive rehabilitation following the acute event is provided. The post-acute healthcare context also refers to the period of time that begins and ends with the initial comprehensive rehabilitation phase, which can vary in different settings. The ICF Core Sets for the post-acute context for neurological, cardiopulmonary and musculoskeletal conditions as well as for patients with spinal cord injury and for geriatric patients are intended for use by physicians, nurses, therapists and other health professionals specialized in rehabilitation or geriatric care provision. At this stage, all potentially relevant aspects of a patient's functioning and relevant Environmental Factors should be taken into account in order to reach an optimal level of functioning. In the post-acute context, ICF Core Sets provide a framework for standardized reports and facilitate the assessment of functioning from a patient-centred and interdisciplinary perspective.[28]

3.2.3. ICF Core Sets for Long-Term Healthcare Context

The long-term healthcare context is the period during which persons with a health condition live in the community and receive both medical and non-medical care intermittently. The ICF Core Sets for the long-term context are health condition related and have been developed for a range of burdensome chronic health conditions. These ICF Core Sets are intended for use in the community-oriented, late phase of rehabilitation and in the community.[34] Since in particular community-oriented care may involve not only health professionals but also experts in other fields, such as social work, as well as employers, family and friends, it is essential that discussions of a patient's problems and needs are understandable to all. For this reason, the standard and common language provided by the ICF Core Sets is of special importance for the long-term healthcare context. In addition, at this stage of care, Environmental Factors play a major role in the patient's integration in the community and the ICF Core Sets draw attention to these environmental influences.

3.2.4. Context Cross-Cutting ICF Core Sets

As with all ICF Core Sets, context cross-cutting ICF Core Sets can be applied in isolation or in combination with other ICF Core Sets as well. The ICF Core Set for Vocational Rehabilitation (VR) is an example.[60] One important aspect of community integration of patients is return to work or participation in a work setting, and VR is an interdisciplinary approach that seeks to optimize work participation and reintegration. The ICF Core Set for VR serves as an international standard of what to measure and report for individuals in VR programs. Applicable to post-acute settings as well as in the long-term context, the ICF Core Set for VR provides a common language for clinicians, researchers, insurers and policymakers in the implementation of VR programmes.

3.3. Types of ICF Core Sets

There are three types of ICF Core Sets: the Comprehensive and Brief ICF Core Sets and the Generic Set. These are described below.

3.3.1. Comprehensive ICF Core Set

The Comprehensive ICF Core Set includes those ICF categories that reflect the entire spectrum of typical problems that persons with a health condition, or in a specific healthcare context, may face. It can serve as a checklist to guide practitioners through assessment so as not to overlook aspects of functioning that are likely to present a problem for a patient. Due to its extensive range of categories, the Comprehensive ICF Core Set is a tool that allows for a thorough and interdisciplinary assessment of functioning for a person with a health condition.

3.3.2. Brief ICF Core Set

The Brief ICF Core Set is derived from the Comprehensive ICF Core Set and is composed of those ICF categories that should be taken into account for any patient with a health condition or in any healthcare context for which the ICF Core Set was developed, and captures the essence of person's experience of functioning and disability. Hence, the Brief ICF Core Set is used when only a brief assessment of functioning is necessary (for example in primary care or a single-discipline setting). It therefore serves as the starting point for condition- or context-related basic clinical documentation. In addition, the Brief ICF Core Set was developed to be used as the minimal standard for efficiently describing functioning and disability in clinical and epidemiological studies.

3.3.3. Generic Set

Unlike the approach used in developing the other ICF Core Sets, the Generic Set was developed from a psychometrics study.[61] The set of seven ICF categories contained in the Generic Set are the categories that best differentiate the different levels of functioning among persons with any health condition in any healthcare context.

The Generic Set is of importance for health statistics and public health. It can be used to compare functioning across health conditions, settings, contexts, countries and population groups using only a small number of ICF categories that are key indicators of health and functioning. The Generic Set is also valuable for clinical use as it depicts the very core of functioning and provides, at a glance, initial insight into a patient's level of functioning that is clear and understandable to any health or health-related professional involved. Most importantly, the Generic Set ensures comparability across health conditions. Because of this, when using any of the other ICF Core Sets it is important to always also use the Generic Set. When it is used on its own it provides a useful summary of information about functioning and can be written on the first page of a patient's medical history to offer a quick overview of the patient's level of functioning.

As one can see, the application of ICF Core Sets is quite versatile. Essential to the optimal application of ICF Core Sets is a decision about the purpose for which they will be used. Knowing the purpose will facilitate the selection of the suitable ICF Core Set(s) to use.

Summary Box

- ICF Core Sets are tools to implement the ICF in clinical practice.
- ICF Core Sets should be used jointly with the ICD.
- 31 ICF Core Sets are currently available for different health conditions and healthcare contexts.
- The three types of ICF Core Sets are: Comprehensive, Brief and Generic.
- When using any ICF Core Set, the Generic Set should also be used for comparability of information.
- ICF Core Sets support the interdisciplinary, comprehensive assessment of functioning.
- To be able to optimally use the ICF Core Sets, it is important to decide on the purpose of their use.

4 Use of ICF Core Sets in Clinical Practice

Alexandra Rauch, Miriam Lückenkemper and Alarcos Cieza

In practice, the ICF Core Sets are tools for describing functioning. Information about a person's functioning is at the core of any clinical assessment, assignment to health services, health interventions, planning and performing of interventions and outcome evaluation. In clinical practice, the ICF Core Sets help to standardize and structure the description of functioning and, as a result, to guide the assessment. Any information gathered in clinical settings using the ICF Core Sets can be aggregated and used for other purposes, such as research, health reporting or health statistics.

The ICF Core Sets have been developed for several health conditions and condition groups, as well as for health service contexts. A total of 31 ICF Core Sets are available, each in a Comprehensive and Brief version. To apply ICF Core Sets in practice, users must select the most appropriate ICF Core Set and then describe the level of functioning. Both steps are introduced in this chapter.

4.1. The Selection of ICF Core Sets ("What to Describe")

The selection of the appropriate ICF Core Set depends on the user's purposes in describing functioning. Users can choose among ICF Core Sets for *specific health-conditions* or *condition groups*. Users should also take into account the healthcare context in which the description is being performed. In addition, users need to select the appropriate *type* of ICF Core Set – Comprehensive or Brief – in light of the amount of information they require to describe the level of functioning for their purpose. As explained further below, the Generic Set should always be included in any description of functioning.

4.1.1. Selection of ICF Core Sets for Particular Health Conditions or Condition Groups

To describe functioning in persons with health conditions, the healthcare context in which the description will take place has to be considered, that is, the context in the continuum of care that is provided to a person. While for acute and post-acute care ICF Core Sets exist for some condition groups (neurological, musculoskeletal, cardiopulmonary) and for acute inflammatory arthritis, ICF Core Sets for specific health conditions have only been developed for long-term care. Thus, the state of the disease, injury or disorder has to be considered when selecting the appropriate ICF Core Set. For example, to describe the functioning of a person with traumatic brain injury (TBI), both the health condition-related *ICF Core Set for TBI*[32] and the condition group-related *ICF Core Sets for Neurological Conditions in Acute Care*[27] and *in Post-Acute Care*[29] – both of which cover TBI – are available. To apply an ICF Core Set to a person with TBI during comprehensive rehabilitation in a specialized rehabilitation facility, for example two years after the injury, the *ICF Core Set for TBI* should be selected (Figure 5). To apply an ICF Core Set to a person in the acute state shortly after the head injury, the condition group-related *ICF Core Set for Neurological Conditions in Acute Care* is more appropriate.

On the other hand, if a person is admitted to a highly specialized acute or post-acute facility, practitioners may wish to select the ICF Core Set for the particular

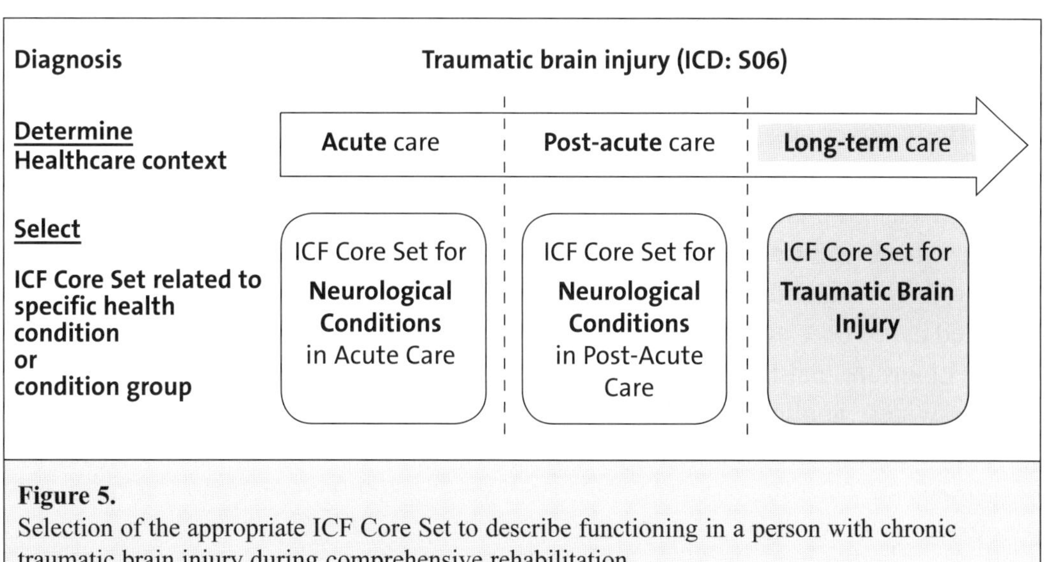

Figure 5.
Selection of the appropriate ICF Core Set to describe functioning in a person with chronic traumatic brain injury during comprehensive rehabilitation

health condition. For example, for a person with acute cardiac infarction due to coronary heart disease who has been admitted to a specialized cardiac centre, the *ICF Core Set for Chronic Ischaemic Heart Disease*[37] can be applied to both the acute and post-acute contexts.

The ICF Core Sets for each condition group take account of the different health conditions in that condition group. For example, the ICF Core Sets for Neurological Conditions in Acute Care[27] and Post-Acute Care[29] include the following diseases and injuries: diseases of the nervous system, head injuries, cerebrovascular diseases, cancer (with impairment of the central nervous system) and lesion of the spinal cord. The ICF Core Sets for Neurological Conditions in Acute Care or Post-Acute Care should be selected only when they relate to these specific diseases and injuries.

4.1.2. Selection of the Type of ICF Core Set

After selecting the appropriate ICF Core Set to describe functioning in a person with a particular health condition, the *type* of ICF Core Set needs to be chosen. There are three types of ICF Core Set: the Generic, Brief and Comprehensive, which vary in the number and specificity of ICF categories included. The selection of the appropriate type depends very much on the setting in which the ICF Core Set will be used and for what purpose. The following considerations can help the user to select the most appropriate type of ICF Core Set:

Generic Set

The Generic Set is composed of seven 2nd level categories from the ICF components Body Functions and Activities and Participation which have been statistically determined to be generally applicable across health conditions and healthcare contexts. As such, the Generic Set can be used for a very brief description of functioning, for example, for population health statistics. Because of its general applicability, it is strongly recommended that the ICF categories from the Generic Set should be included every time another type of ICF Core Set, Brief or Comprehensive, is used. This will ensure that the data collected in a clinical setting for assessment purposes has the widest applicability for other purposes, including health statistics, health services planning and research.

Brief ICF Core Set

Brief ICF Core Sets consist of categories from all of the ICF components selected from the corresponding Comprehensive ICF Core Sets. As mentioned, in practice when a Brief ICF Core Set is used, the Generic Set should also be used. Categories included in the Brief ICF Core Set are taken only from the 2nd or 1st level, so they are used for a broader and less detailed description of functioning. They are used to describe only the most likely areas of functioning associated with a health condition, as well as those areas for which information is required. Brief ICF Core Sets are most useful for describing functioning from the perspective of a single healthcare provider setting, but can also be used in interdisciplinary teams. The amount of information about functioning included in a Brief ICF Core Set may also be helpful to inform professionals working in other settings or health insurers for service planning.

Enlarged Brief version: Brief Core Set augmented with selected categories from the Comprehensive ICF Core Set

The use of Brief ICF Core Sets facilitates a broad description of functioning that offers professionals, in particular those working in a single discipline health facility, a starting point for the description of functioning in persons with specific health

Table 6.
Example from chapter "d4 Mobility": Selection of additional ICF categories from the Comprehensive ICF Core Sets for Spinal Cord Injury to augment the Brief ICF Core Set to the Enlarged Brief version

Brief ICF Core Set		Enlarged Brief version = Additional categories	
d410	Changing basic body positions	d410	Changing basic body positions
		d4103**	**Sitting**
		d4104**	**Standing**
		d415*	**Maintaining a body position**
d420	Transferring oneself	d420	Transferring oneself
d445	Hand and arm use	d445	Hand and arm use
d450	Walking	d450	Walking
		d4501**	**Walking short distances**
		d4502**	**Walking long distances**

* Selection of additional category; ** Selection of a more specific category

conditions. If additional areas of functioning or more detailed specification of categories from the 3rd or 4th level are required to describe functioning adequately, a user can select categories from the corresponding Comprehensive ICF Core Set and then add them to the Brief ICF Core Set. The result can be called a "Enlarged Brief" Core Set. For example, a physical therapist may choose the Brief ICF Core Set for Spinal Cord Injury in Post-Acute Care but finds that he or she needs more precise information about mobility. The therapist can choose additional categories or more specific categories from the Comprehensive ICF Core Set to describe the information that is needed, as shown in Table 6.

Comprehensive ICF Core Set

Comprehensive ICF Core Sets should be used for a complete and detailed description of functioning. We recommend that whenever the Comprehensive ICF Core Set is used, the ICF categories from the Generic Set that are not included in the Comprehensive Core Set, be added. In some cases, a Comprehensive ICF Core Set includes more than 100 categories from the 1st chapter level to the 4th category level, so applying a Comprehensive ICF Core Set for the description of functioning can be time-consuming. Because of this, Comprehensive ICF Core Sets are most useful in interdisciplinary settings for which an exhaustive description of functioning can be distributed among team members from different professions, as in interdisciplinary assessment for rehabilitation planning. Comprehensive ICF Core Sets can also be used as a reference for describing functioning to guide users through the assessment process and to remind them not to overlook categories of functioning that are likely to present a problem for a person with a particular health condition.

For example, during an interdisciplinary rehabilitation programme for a person in a chronic state after a traumatic brain injury (TBI), the interdisciplinary team needs to identify the person's rehabilitation needs for comprehensive intervention planning. Therefore, the Comprehensive ICF Core Set for TBI was selected (see Figure 6).

Additional options: When a person experiences multiple health conditions, it is possible to combine several ICF Core Sets or to pick ICF categories from other ICF Core Sets and add them to the ICF Core Set for the main health condition. In many situations, the Enlarged Brief version may be the most feasible solution for applying ICF Core Sets in practice.

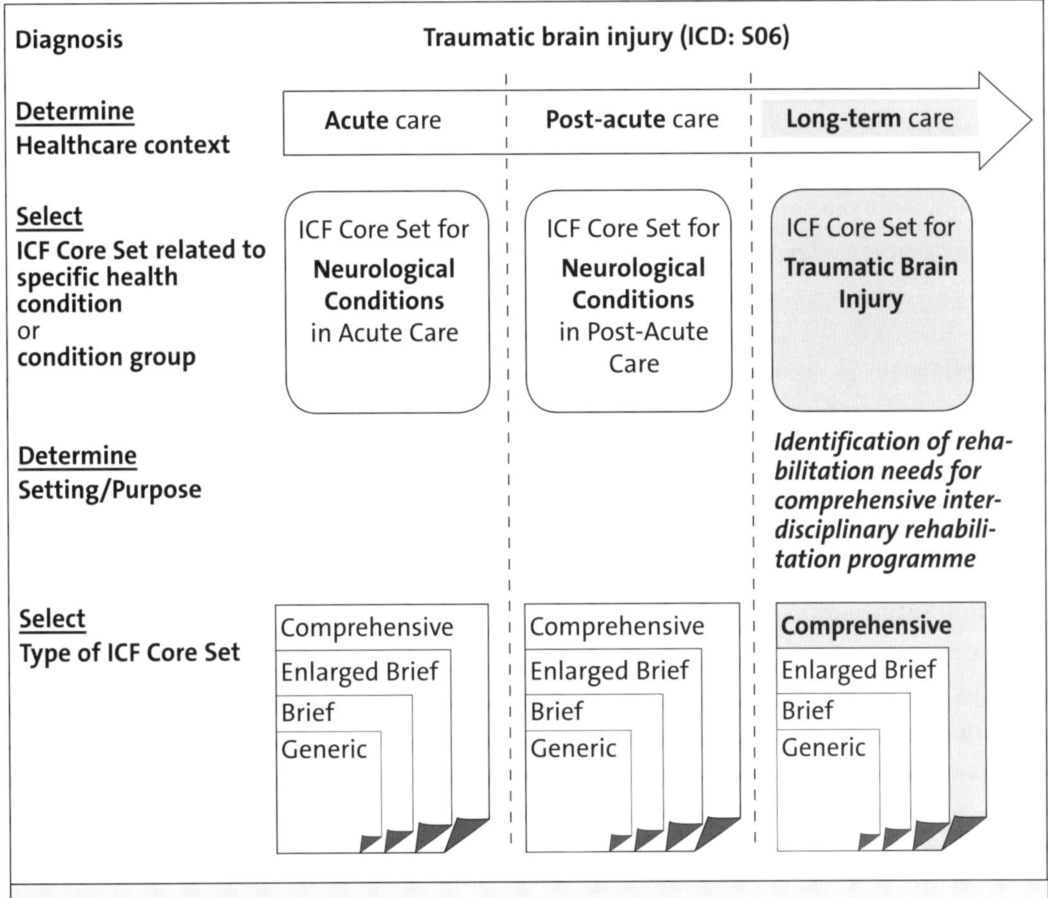

Figure 6.
Selection of the type of ICF Core Sets to identify rehabilitation needs in a person with chronic traumatic brain injury for comprehensive interdisciplinary rehabilitation

4.2. The Description of the Level of Functioning ("How to Describe")

Once the appropriate ICF Core Set is selected, it is then possible to create a profile of functioning for the patient. Usually this requires appropriate assessment. ICF categories are the building blocks of ICF Core Sets and provide a list of those areas of functioning that need to be assessed. Each category in the ICF is defined with inclusions and exclusions that help to operationalize the category for use.

4.2.1. Sources of Information

Once the meaning of the ICF category is clear, the user should gather relevant information about each ICF category. Only by means of a comprehensive picture of a person's level of functioning in different domains appropriate person-centred intervention planning can be performed. In clinical practice, the following sources of information to describe functioning can be used where available.

Case History

A case history is usually performed during the initial contact between the responsible professional and a patient, although it may be repeated over the course of the treatment process. The case history gathers verbal information from an interview with the patient, the patient's family members, caregivers or other proxy sources. In addition, information can be extracted from patient records or other documentation. A case history combines the patient's perspective of his or her level of functioning with objective information. The use of an ICF Core Set can guide professionals through the process of case history taking so that they describe all relevant areas of functioning from both the patient's and the health professional's perspectives.

Patient-Reported Questionnaires

Patient-reported questionnaires are used to obtain information from the patient's perspective in a written and standardized form. Their use for assessment can contribute to a better understanding of the experience of functioning for persons with health conditions. Such questionnaires can ask about quality of life, e.g. SF36 (Short Form Medical Outcomes Study 36 Health Survey);[62] specific functions such as hand and arm functions, e.g. DASH (Disability of the Arm, Shoulder and Hand);[63] walking, e.g. Walking Impairment Questionnaire;[64] about general levels of functioning in persons with specific health conditions such as with low back pain (Oswestry Disability Questionnaire[65]), osteoarthritis (Western Ontario and McMaster Universities Osteoarthritis Index, WOMAC[66]) or depression (Beck Depression Inventory[67]).

The information obtained from questionnaires can be used to evaluate the extent of the problem in the components of functioning or the extent of barrier or facilitator in the Environmental Factors in different ways. Single items included in a questionnaire can be used to generate information to describe an ICF category. For example, the question from the SF36 "*Did you have a lot of energy?*" provides information to describe ICF category *b130 Energy and drive.* The information of subscales of questionnaires can also be used. For example, the work module of the DASH combines four questions related to problems at work, namely: "*Did you have any difficulty in…*" (1) "*…using your usual technique for your work?*", (2) "*…doing your usual work because of arm, shoulder or hand pain?*", (3) "*…doing your work as well as you would like?*", and (4) "*…spending your usual amount of time doing your work?*" This subscale is valuable as it can be used to describe the level of functioning in *d850 Remunerative employment.* In the same way an entire questionnaire can be used to describe functioning in an ICF category. For example, to describe *d450 Walking* in a person with peripheral arterial disease, the information provided by the complete Walking Impairment Questionnaire can be used as the basis for the description of the level of functioning.

Clinical Examination

Clinical examinations are usually performed by experts in distinct areas of functioning. The examinations are frequently performed using standardized measures such as:

- single item standardized measures assessing one domain of functioning, such as blood pressure using a blood pressure cuff, body temperature using a clinical thermometer, muscle power using manual muscle testing, joint mobility using a goniometer or walking by measuring walking distance on a treadmill.
- comprehensive standardized measures assessing a combination of different domains of functioning such as different cognitive functions in the Mini-Mental State Examination,[68] independence in various daily activities in the Barthel Index,[69] or diverse motor functions in the Rivermead Mobility Index.[70] The translation of items obtained from comprehensive standardized measures to ICF categories is based on the same intuitive principles as in the patient reported questionnaires.

For ICF categories for which there are no standardized measures or for which patient statements are unavailable, visual inspections or observations may provide an alternative source of information. Moreover, in practice, observations are sometimes preferred because standardized measures are often too time-consuming. Although the description of the problem based on observation is a matter of clinical judgment and experience, it still allows a reasonable evaluation of a problem. For example, to identify a person's problem in *d455 Moving around*, the health professional may observe the person in different situations (running, climbing, skipping, etc.) and evaluate the person's capacity and performance in doing these tasks.

Technical Investigation

In addition to clinical examinations, technical investigations, including diagnostic procedures, are performed using specialized equipment such as magnetic resonance imaging (MRI), radiographs, ultrasound imaging or electromyography. In some cases, appropriate equipment is not available although it is needed to make a clinical determination (in low resource countries, for example, there may be no X-ray machine to test for fractures). In these cases there may be too little information to allow an adequate description of a specific area of functioning (*s7700 Bones* in this case).

To facilitate the assignment of items included in patient-reported questionnaires or derived from clinical examination or technical investigation to ICF categories, existing linking rules can be applied.[71–72]

4.2.2. Description of the Problem

Assessment

It is important to document the results of assessment for intervention planning, clinical monitoring, outcome evaluation and other purposes. However, resulting information may be too discipline-specific and, therefore, too difficult to be understood by professionals who are not experts in that field. For example, not all members of an interdisciplinary team will understand what a value of "3" on the Manual Muscle Testing Scale means. In such cases a more general description of a person's level of disability may facilitate the information exchange among the same or different professionals and possibly across different levels of the health system. To evaluate the degree of a disability, the ICF qualifiers can be used as a general rating scale.

Using the ICF Qualifiers

The qualifier system of the ICF can be applied as a summary or global evaluation of information gathered concerning specific areas of functioning. The existing information from the assessment of functioning is the basis for the application of ICF qualifiers. In most cases, the ICF qualifiers are used for all ICF categories at the 2nd and more detailed levels. In some ICF Core Sets, they are also applied to the 1st level (chapters) and to blocks. The rating of chapters and blocks may be a challenge for clinicians as information about different specific domains of functioning has to be aggregated into a single value of the ICF qualifier. Based on the available information, the level (and in Body Structures also the nature and location) of disability can be rated for each ICF category with at least one or up to four ICF qualifiers. As a minimum, the first qualifier is used in all components. To provide more information, additional qualifiers can be used depending on the component:

In practice, users are advised to use the first qualifier (extent of impairment) for Body Functions and the first (extent of impairment), second (nature of impairment) and third qualifier (location of impairment) for Body Structures. However, the second and third qualifiers in Body Structures should only be applied if impairment exists at all.

Activities and Participation has two qualifiers, the first (performance) and second (capacity). In order to have a meaningful description of capacity, the question is what we consider assistance in the description of capacity or not. When the type of assistance consists of a physical change in the body, as in the implantation of devices such as a pacemaker, an internal hip prosthesis or artificial internal lenses for the eye, the result should not be viewed as assistance as these interventions actually change the person's intrinsic capacity level for a domain of functioning. So in a person with a newly implanted artificial hip joint, walking capacity should be rated in terms of the enhanced capacity made possible by the artificial hip joint. On the other hand, when the type of assistance is outside of the body, as in devices such as splints, crutches, wheelchairs, specialized computer technology or environmental control units, capacity should be rated without considering the impact of these facilitating devices (see the example in Figure 7 below).

The rating of Environmental Factors is performed with the first qualifier to describe facilitators or barriers. In some cases, one and the same Environmental Factor can both be a facilitator and a barrier. For example, the use of *e1101 Drugs* (e.g. pain killers) can reduce problems in some Body Functions (e.g. *b280 Sensation of Pain*), but cause problems in the form of side effects in other Body Functions (e.g. *b5350 Sensation of nausea*).

Using the qualifiers to rate the extent of difficulty is not governed by rules set out in the ICF but is left entirely to the clinical experience of the rater once he or she has considered all available information.

4.3. The Documentation Form

To facilitate the description of functioning using ICF Core Sets in practice, a documentation form has been prepared that integrates all areas of information necessary for the description of functioning using the ICF Core Sets (see Figure 7). This documentation form includes all steps described above. The structure of the documentation form provides the following properties and entry options:

① The **categories** included in the ICF Core Set to be used. Each ICF category is represented with code and title. The form also includes the definition of each ICF category (for all components except Body Structures). If available, inclusions and exclusions are given. Depending on the ICF Core Set, the documentation form may contain 2nd to 4th-level categories or, for some of the ICF Core Sets, blocks or chapters as well.

② The **source of available information** used for the description of the problem can be marked by checking the options "Case history", "Patient-reported questionnaires", "Clinical examination" or "Technical investigation".

③ Space is provided for the **description of the problem**, which facilitates the documentation of assessment results. This field allows the documentation of the results of a case history, questionnaire, clinical examination or technical investigation in free text or narrative form. In Activites and Participation, capacity and performance are described separately.

④ Columns for indicating the **ICF qualifier** describing the extent of the problem (0–4, respectively 0–7, 8 and 9) are provided for each category. Depending on which component they belong to, one, two or three qualifiers can be applied for rating: the extent of the impairment in Body Functions, the extent, nature and location of impairment in Body Structures, performance and capacity in Activities and Participation, and the extent of a facilitator or barrier in Environmental Factors.

The documentation forms for the Comprehensive and Brief ICF Core Sets always include the additional ICF categories from the Generic Set unless these categories were already in the ICF Core Sets. In some cases, an ICF category of the Generic Set and a category of a Comprehensive ICF Core Set are part of the same ICF domain but are at different hierarchical levels. In such cases all categories from all levels are included in the documentation form and will be rated by an ICF qualifier. For example, the domain walking is covered by the 2nd-level category *d450 Walking* in the Generic Set, but the Comprehensive ICF Core Set for Spinal Cord Injury in Post-Acute Care contains the more detailed 3rd-level categories *d4500 Walking short distances*, *d4501 Walking long distances*, *d4502 Walking on different surfaces* and *d4503 Walking around obstacles*. Here, all information from the 3rd-level categories has to be integrated to come up with a single value in order to be able to rate the 2nd-level category. The inclusion of all categories from the Generic Set ensures the availability of information for health reporting, which is the main purpose of the Generic Set.

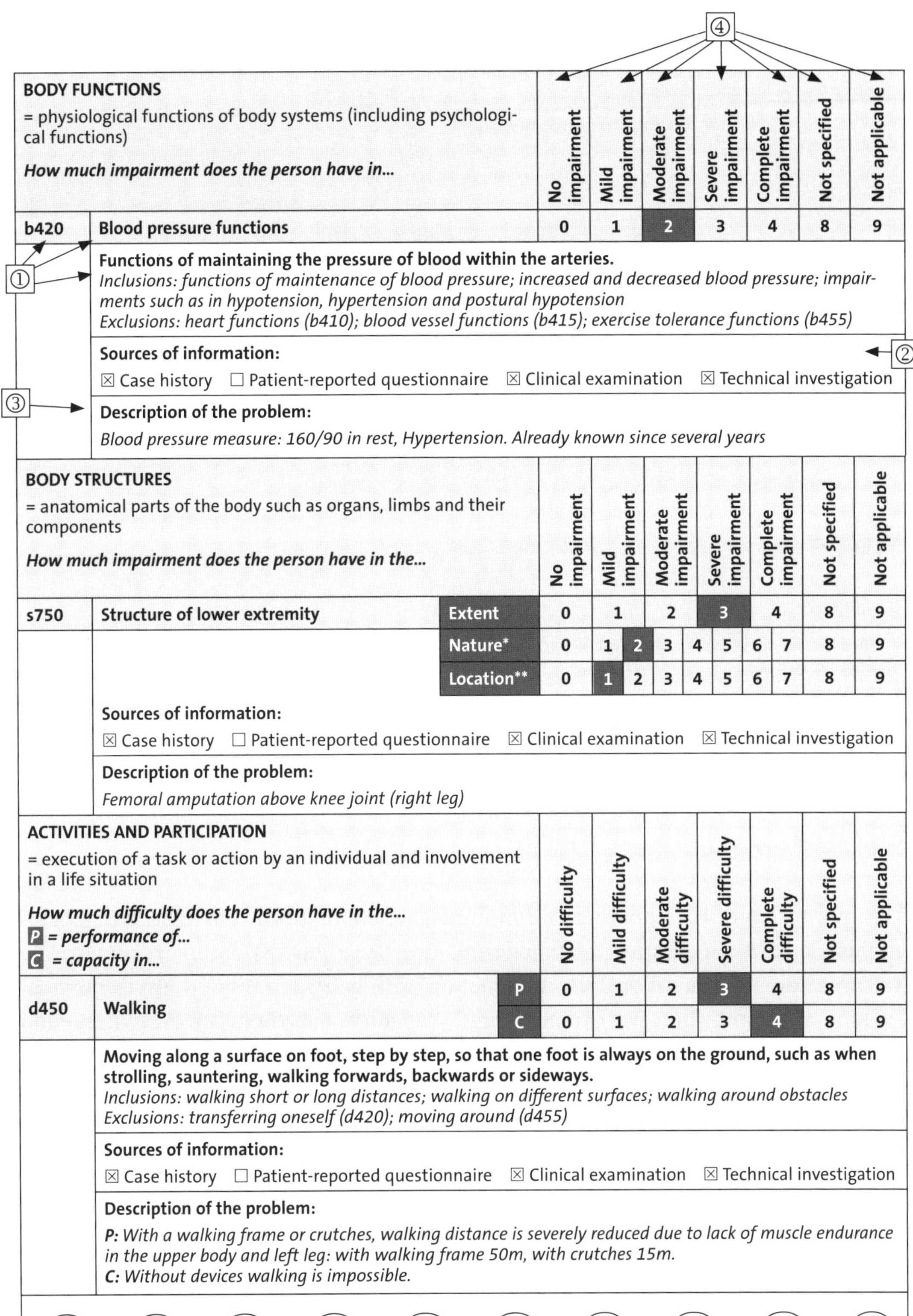

BODY FUNCTIONS = physiological functions of body systems (including psychological functions) ***How much impairment does the person have in...***		No impairment	Mild impairment	Moderate impairment	Severe impairment	Complete impairment	Not specified	Not applicable
b420	Blood pressure functions	0	1	**2**	3	4	8	9

Functions of maintaining the pressure of blood within the arteries.
Inclusions: functions of maintenance of blood pressure; increased and decreased blood pressure; impairments such as in hypotension, hypertension and postural hypotension
Exclusions: heart functions (b410); blood vessel functions (b415); exercise tolerance functions (b455)

Sources of information:
☒ Case history ☐ Patient-reported questionnaire ☒ Clinical examination ☒ Technical investigation

Description of the problem:
Blood pressure measure: 160/90 in rest, Hypertension. Already known since several years

BODY STRUCTURES = anatomical parts of the body such as organs, limbs and their components ***How much impairment does the person have in the...***			No impairment	Mild impairment		Moderate impairment		Severe impairment		Complete impairment		Not specified	Not applicable
s750	Structure of lower extremity	Extent	0	1		2		**3**		4		8	9
		Nature*	0	1	**2**	3	4	5	6	7		8	9
		Location**	0	**1**	2	3	4	5	6	7		8	9

Sources of information:
☒ Case history ☐ Patient-reported questionnaire ☒ Clinical examination ☒ Technical investigation

Description of the problem:
Femoral amputation above knee joint (right leg)

ACTIVITIES AND PARTICIPATION = execution of a task or action by an individual and involvement in a life situation ***How much difficulty does the person have in the...*** ***P = performance of...*** ***C = capacity in...***			No difficulty	Mild difficulty	Moderate difficulty	Severe difficulty	Complete difficulty	Not specified	Not applicable
d450	Walking	P	0	1	2	**3**	4	8	9
		C	0	1	2	3	**4**	8	9

Moving along a surface on foot, step by step, so that one foot is always on the ground, such as when strolling, sauntering, walking forwards, backwards or sideways.
Inclusions: walking short or long distances; walking on different surfaces; walking around obstacles
Exclusions: transferring oneself (d420); moving around (d455)

Sources of information:
☒ Case history ☐ Patient-reported questionnaire ☒ Clinical examination ☒ Technical investigation

Description of the problem:
P: *With a walking frame or crutches, walking distance is severely reduced due to lack of muscle endurance in the upper body and left leg: with walking frame 50m, with crutches 15m.*
C: *Without devices walking is impossible.*

Figure 7. Continued on next page

ENVIRONMENTAL FACTORS = make up the physical, social and attitudinal environment in which people live and conduct their lives ***How much of a facilitator or barrier does the person experience with respect to...***		Complete facilitator	Substantial facilitator	Moderate facilitator	Mild facilitator	No barrier/facilitator	Mild barrier	Moderate barrier	Substantial barrier	Complete barrier	Not specified	Not applicable
e120	**Products and technology for personal indoor and outdoor mobility and transportation**	**+4**	**+3**	**+2**	**+1**	**0**	**1**	**2**	**3**	**4**	**8**	**9**
	Equipment, products and technologies used by people in activities of moving inside and outside buildings, including those adapted or specially designed, located in, on or near the person using them. *Inclusions: general and assistive products and technology for personal indoor and outdoor mobility and transportation*											
	Sources of information: ☒ Case history ☐ Patient-reported questionnaire ☒ Clinical examination ☒ Technical investigation											
	Description of the facilitator/barrier: *Walking frame and crutches have been adapted. Toilet chair on loan.*											

Figure 7
The documentation form (extraction from the ICF Core Set for Musculoskeletal Conditions in Acute Care)

* Rating of the nature of the impairment in Body Structures: 0 = no change in structure, 1 = total absence, 2 = partial absence, 3 = additional part, 4 = aberrant dimension, 5 = discontinuity, 6 = deviating position, 7 = qualitative changes in structure, 8 = not specified, 9 = not applicable
** Rating of the location of the impairment in Body Structures: 0 = more than one region, 1 = right, 2 = left, 3 = both sides, 4 = front, 5 = back, 6 = proximal, 7 = distal, 8 = not specified, 9 = not applicable

Creating a Functioning Profile

The application of ICF qualifiers for rating the extent of a problem in each ICF category is the basis for creating the functioning profile (Figure 8). A functioning profile illustrates the first qualifier in Body Functions, Body Structures and Environmental Factors and both the performance and capacity qualifiers in Activities and Participation. This identifies the impact of the environment on level of functioning.

A functioning profile illustrates the levels of functioning across the domains included in the ICF Core Set and thus facilitates the illustration of a person's overall lived experience of health in relation to his or her health condition.

For all ICF Core Sets, blank documentation forms and functioning profiles are provided on a CD accompanying this manual.

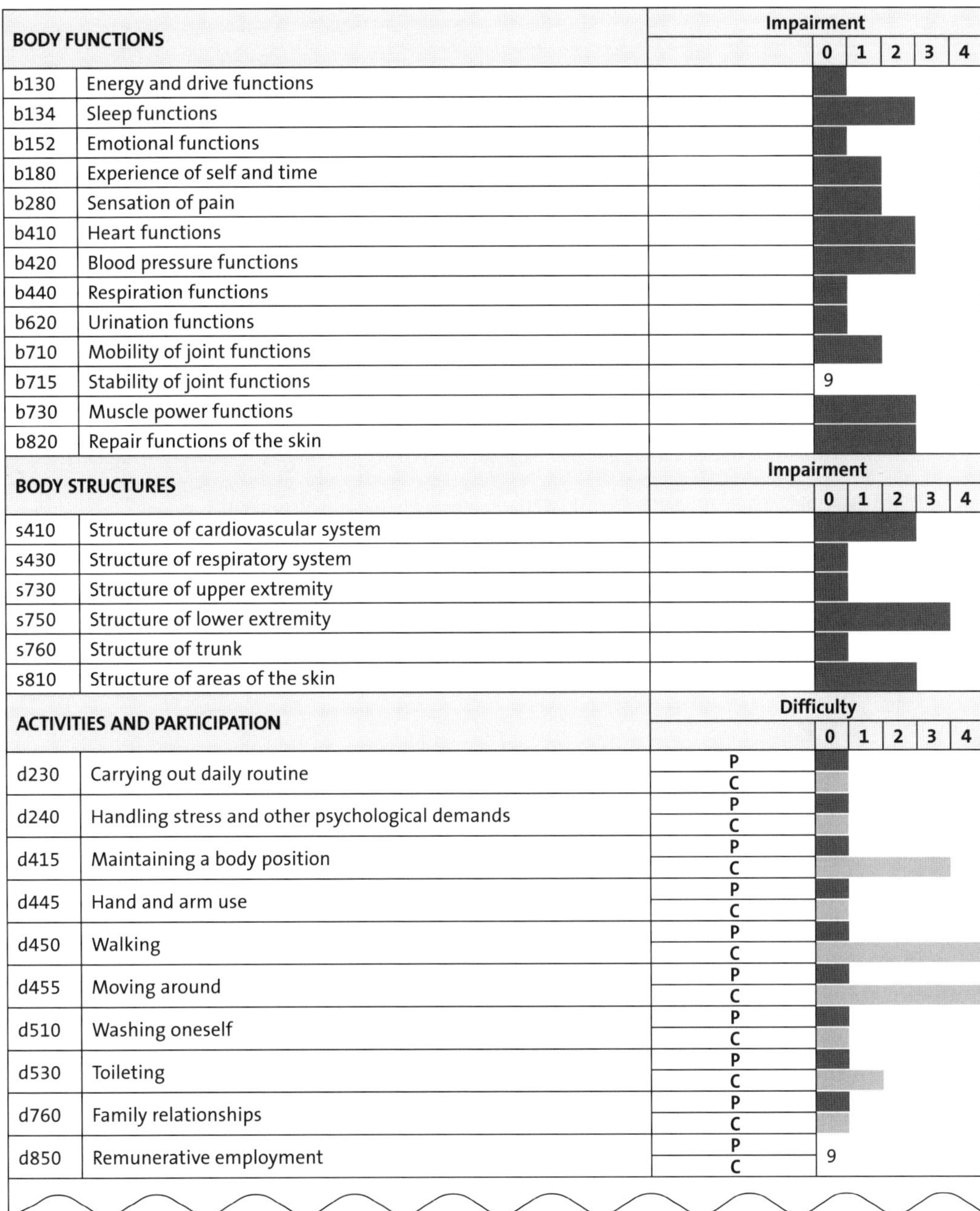

BODY FUNCTIONS		Impairment 0 1 2 3 4
b130	Energy and drive functions	
b134	Sleep functions	
b152	Emotional functions	
b180	Experience of self and time	
b280	Sensation of pain	
b410	Heart functions	
b420	Blood pressure functions	
b440	Respiration functions	
b620	Urination functions	
b710	Mobility of joint functions	
b715	Stability of joint functions	9
b730	Muscle power functions	
b820	Repair functions of the skin	

BODY STRUCTURES		Impairment 0 1 2 3 4
s410	Structure of cardiovascular system	
s430	Structure of respiratory system	
s730	Structure of upper extremity	
s750	Structure of lower extremity	
s760	Structure of trunk	
s810	Structure of areas of the skin	

ACTIVITIES AND PARTICIPATION			Difficulty 0 1 2 3 4
d230	Carrying out daily routine	P / C	
d240	Handling stress and other psychological demands	P / C	
d415	Maintaining a body position	P / C	
d445	Hand and arm use	P / C	
d450	Walking	P / C	
d455	Moving around	P / C	
d510	Washing oneself	P / C	
d530	Toileting	P / C	
d760	Family relationships	P / C	
d850	Remunerative employment	P / C	9

Figure 8. Continued on next page

ENVIRONMENTAL FACTORS		Facilitator					Barrier			
		+4	+3	+2	+1	0	1	2	3	4
e110	Products or substances for personal consumption									
e120	Products and techn. for pers. indoor and outdoor mobility and transportation									
e310	Immediate family									
e355	Health professionals									
e410	Individual attitudes of immediate family members									
e580	Health services, systems and policies									

Figure 8.
Functioning profile (extraction from ICF Core Set for Spinal Cord Injury in Post-Acute Care)

In Body Functions, Body Structures, Activities and Participation: 0 = no problem, 1 = mild problem, 2 = moderate problem, 3 = severe problem, 4 = complete problem; In Environmental Factors: 0 = no barrier/facilitator, 1 = mild barrier, 2 = moderate barrier, 3 = severe barrier, 4 = complete barrier, +1 = mild facilitator, +2 = moderate facilitator, +3 = substantial facilitator, +4 = complete facilitator

P = Performance, C = Capacity

Summary Box

Selection of the appropriate ICF Core Set

- ICF Core Sets are available as *health conditions* or *health condition group* ICF Core Sets depending on the healthcare context and the user's purposes.
- ICF Core Sets for particular health conditions were developed for the long-term context, whereas ICF Core Sets for condition groups were developed for acute and post-acute care.
- ICF Core Sets for *Sleep* and *Hand conditions* are available for long-term care and the ICF Core Set for *Vocational Rehabilitation* extends to all health conditions and healthcare contexts in which vocational rehabilitation is provided.
- There are three types of ICF Core Sets that may be selected: the Generic and the Brief and Comprehensive ICF Core Sets. In addition, it is often useful to augment a Brief ICF Core Set with additional categories from the Comprehensive ICF Core Set, which is the Enlarged Brief version.

Documentation of functioning based on the use of ICF Core Sets

- The *documentation form* provides the framework for describing a patient's problems or strengths for different ICF categories.
- Information for describing the categories is gathered from an assessment.

Different *sources of information* can be used: case history, patient-reported questionnaires, clinical examination and technical investigation.

- Assessment results are rated by the *ICF qualifiers*. Applying ICF qualifiers facilitates the creation of a patient's functioning profile.

The documentation form to create a functioning profile mentioned in this manual is also available in an open access interactive web-based format www.icf-core-sets.org

5 Use Cases

To illustrate the application of ICF Core Sets in practice, this chapter provides five use cases from real persons. These cases arose in the rehabilitation context and focus on the rehabilitative strategy in health care, which emphasizes assessing functioning for the purpose of optimising a person's capacity and strengthening the resources of the individual.[4, 73] The ICF Core Sets can be used for other health strategies and indeed intervention strategies outside of the realm of health in social, employment and educational contexts, but rehabilitation applications provide clear use cases for the purposes of this manual. Each of the following cases focuses on a health condition and, in addition, highlights a theme relevant for the practical application of the ICF Core Sets. The following table provides an overview of the use cases and their themes:

Use Case 1: ICF Core Set for Musculoskeletal Conditions in Acute Care

Theme: Applying ICF Core Sets in persons with several health conditions

Use Case 2: ICF Core Set for Spinal Cord Injury in Post-Acute Care

Theme: Applying ICF Core Sets in multidisciplinary settings

Use Case 3: ICF Core Set for Multiple Sclerosis

Theme: Considering patient's resources in ICF Core Set-based documentation

Use Case 4: ICF Core Set for Vocational Rehabilitation

Theme: Describing and differentiating between capacity and performance

Use Case 5: ICF Core Set for Low Back Pain

Theme: Representing detailed clinical information using an ICF Core Set

5.1. Use Case 1: Applying the ICF Core Set for Musculoskeletal Conditions in Acute Care

Alexandra Rauch

This use case illustrates the application of an ICF Core Set to a patient who had a leg amputated due to vascular disease and now receives postoperative care in the acute unit of a hospital. The case also discusses the challenges in the selection of appropriate ICF Core Sets for persons with several health conditions for application in clinical practice.

5.1.1. The Case

Mr. Miller, a 68 year old widowed man, has suffered from peripheral arterial obstructive disease (pAOD) for many years. He also has diabetes mellitus and arterial hypertension and has artificial aortic and mitral valves that are insufficient (Grade 1). One year ago, bypass surgery was performed because of severe vascular undersupply in the right leg related to the pAOD. Unfortunately, the symptoms related to the pAOD have increased again in the last weeks. Two weeks ago, discomfort increased rapidly with severe pain in the right lower leg and related incremental reduction of walking capacity. Mr. Miller's general practitioner admitted him to hospital because of the presumed severe vascular undersupply. Immediate technical investigations showed an acute occlusion of the bypass caused by a thrombosis in the right leg. The evaluation of the results of the clinical examination and technical investigation indicated that a transfemoral amputation above the knee joint was necessary. Since the surgery seven days ago, the patient has been treated in the acute unit of the hospital.

5.1.2. The Application Area and Setting

This acute unit of the hospital is specialized for the treatment of vascular diseases. Several surgeons perform a variety of vascular surgeries on a daily routine. In the acute unit, the management of the consequences of amputations focuses on post-operative treatment. Patients who have undergone amputation normally are discharged home or to a rehabilitation facility as soon as their health condition has stabilized and wound healing is completed. In this unit, two physical therapists treat patients based on medical prescription. Apart from treating patients, the physical therapists are responsible for reporting the level of functioning, which, in addition to the medical report, are used for treatment planning and discharge planning.

5.1.3. The Purpose of Applying an ICF Core Set

To comprehensively describe the patient's level of functioning, the ICF is applied. The results of this description can serve as the basis for treatment planning and preparing the discharge report that will be sent to the rehabilitation facility.

5.1.4. Selection of the Appropriate ICF Core Set

The selection of the appropriate ICF Core Set is performed in two steps: Selection of the health condition-related or condition group-related ICF Core Set and of the appropriate type of ICF Core Set (Figure 9).

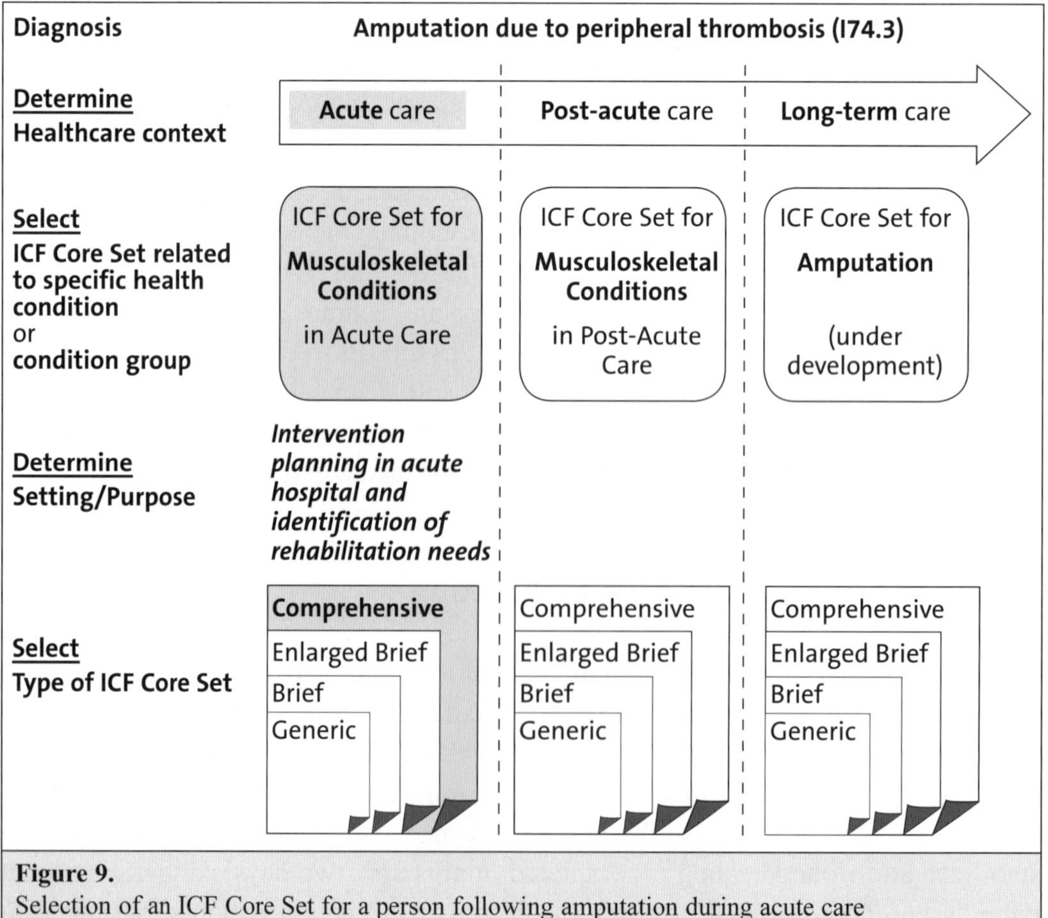

Figure 9.
Selection of an ICF Core Set for a person following amputation during acute care

Choice of ICF Core Set Related to Specific Health Condition or Condition Group

To describe this patient's level of functioning, the *ICF Core Set for Musculoskeletal Conditions in Acute Care*[41, 59, 74] was selected. ICF Core Sets for **acute care** have been developed to facilitate the description of functioning in patients with acute illness or injury and following surgical care.[28] For this health care context, ICF Core Sets have been developed for condition groups instead of specific health conditions (with the exception of acute inflammatory arthritis).

The length of stay in the acute hospital is usually short and the focus is on medical and surgical services. Hence, there is only limited time for rehabilitation interventions that focus on the restoration and maintenance of functioning, the avoidance of complications such as pneumonia, thrombosis, pulmonary embolism, pressure sores and other consequences related to a lack of mobilization.[75] ICF Core Sets for patients in acute care allow physicians, nurses, therapists and other health professionals not specialized in rehabilitation to describe functioning and to integrate this common understanding of functioning for treatment in acute care of a health condition.[28] This facilitates the identification of rehabilitation needs and discharge planning to continue treatment in other rehabilitation facilities.

In this use case, Mr. Miller is suffering from multiple cardiovascular health conditions, although his main diagnosis and the reason for hospital admission was the femoral amputation secondary to pAOD. Thus, to identify and describe the potential problems in functioning related to this acute illness, the *ICF Core Set for* ***Musculoskeletal Conditions*** *in Acute Care* was selected. The following heath conditions are included in this condition group-specific ICF Core Set:

- Multiple trauma
- Fractures of the upper and lower extremities
- Amputations
- Singular musculoskeletal injuries
- Arthropathies (requiring surgery)
- Spine disorders (requiring surgery)

The Comprehensive version of this ICF Core Set [41] consists of 47 2nd-level ICF categories while the Brief[59] includes 27 2nd-level ICF categories.

Choice of Type of ICF Core Set

The selection of the type of ICF Core Set determines the number of ICF categories used for the description of functioning. In this case, the **Comprehensive** ICF Core

Set was selected to allow for the description of a variety of areas of functioning that should be considered for treatment planning and, in particular, to identify Mr. Miller's continuing rehabilitation needs. As noted, it is recommended that all of the ICF categories in the Generic Set not already included in a Comprehensive ICF Core Set be added. In this case, the categories *d230 Carrying out daily routine*, *d455 Moving around*, and *d850 Remunerative employment* from the Generic Set were added to the Comprehensive ICF Core Set for Musculoskeletal Conditions in Acute Care. To address the patient's impairments in Body Functions related to his chronic heart conditions, two additional ICF categories (*b410 Heart functions*, *b420 Blood pressure functions*) from the ICF Core Set for Cardiopulmonary Conditions in Acute Care[35] were also added to the Comprehensive ICF Core Set.

5.1.5. The Description of Functioning with the Documentation Form

To describe Mr. Miller's level of functioning, the documentation form was filled out for the Comprehensive ICF Core Set for Musculoskeletal Conditions in Acute Care, the three additional categories from the Generic Set and the two additional ICF categories selected from the ICF Core Set for Cardiopulmonary Conditions in Acute Care. Information was taken from the case history, previous medical reports, results of technical investigations and a patient interview. Clinical examinations were also performed in several areas of functioning. The resulting information was then rated using the ICF qualifiers based on the clinical experience of the physical therapist. The results of each of these steps were entered in the documentation form (Figure 10) and from this the functioning profile (Figure 11) was created. In these figures, the Brief ICF Core Set for Musculoskeletal Conditions augmented with the Generic Set and the additional two ICF categories are presented; the full version is available in the CD included with the manual.

BODY FUNCTIONS = physiological functions of body systems (including psychological functions) ***How much impairment does the person have in...***		No impairment	Mild impairment	Moderate impairment	Severe impairment	Complete impairment	Not specified	Not applicable
b130	**Energy and drive functions**	**[0]**	1	2	3	4	8	9
	General mental functions of physiological and psychological mechanisms that cause the individual to move towards satisfying specific needs and general goals in a persistent manner. *Inclusions: functions of energy level, motivation, appetite, craving (including craving for substances that can be abused), and impulse control* *Exclusions: consciousness functions (b110); temperament and personality functions (b126); sleep functions (b134); psychomotor functions (b147); emotional functions (b152)*							
	Sources of information: ☒ Case history ☐ Patient-reported questionnaire ☐ Clinical examination ☐ Technical investigation							
	Description of the problem: *Has a lot of energy and motivation to participate in treatment and therapy, is performing exercises on his own.*							
b152	**Emotional functions**	**[0]**	1	2	3	4	8	9
	Specific mental functions related to the feeling and affective components of the processes of the mind. *Inclusions: functions of appropriateness of emotion, regulation and range of emotion; affect; sadness, happiness, love, fear, anger, hate, tension, anxiety, joy, sorrow; lability of emotion; flattening of affect* *Exclusions: temperament and personality functions (b126); energy and drive functions (b130)*							
	Sources of information: ☒ Case history ☐ Patient-reported questionnaire ☐ Clinical examination ☐ Technical investigation							
	Description of the problem: *Is coping with his actual health condition appropriately, no abnormal sadness or emotional instability.*							
b280	**Sensation of pain**	0	**[1]**	2	3	4	8	9
	Sensation of unpleasant feeling indicating potential or actual damage to some body structure. *Inclusions: sensations of generalized or localized pain in one or more body part, pain in a dermatome, stabbing pain, burning pain, dull pain, aching pain; impairments such as myalgia, analgesia and hyperalgesia*							
	Sources of information: ☐ Case history ☐ Patient-reported questionnaire ☒ Clinical examination ☐ Technical investigation							
	Description of the problem: *Visual Analog Scale (VAS, 0-10): 2 in rest and movement; Pain is located in wound area.*							
b410+	**Heart functions**	0	1	**[2]**	3	4	8	9
	Functions of pumping the blood in adequate or required amounts and pressure throughout the body. *Inclusions: functions of heart rate, rhythm and output; contraction force of ventricular muscles; functions of heart valves; pumping the blood through the pulmonary circuit; dynamics of circulation to the heart; impairments such as tachycardia, bradycardia and irregular heart beat and as in heart failure, cardiomyopathy, myocarditis and coronary insufficiency, Exclusions: blood vessel functions (b415); blood pressure functions (b420); exercise tolerance functions (b455)*							
	Sources of information: ☒ Case history ☐ Patient-reported questionnaire ☐ Clinical examination ☐ Technical investigation							
	Description of the problem: *Insufficiency of artificial aortic and mitral valves (grade 1)*							

Figure 10. Continued on next page

b415	**Blood vessel functions**	0	1	2	**3**	4	8	9

Functions of transporting blood throughout the body.
Inclusions: functions of arteries, capillaries and veins; vasomotor function; functions of pulmonary arteries, capillaries and veins; functions of valves of veins; impairments such as in blockage or constriction of arteries; atherosclerosis, arteriosclerosis, thromboembolism and varicose veins
Exclusions: heart functions (b410); blood pressure functions (b420); haematological system functions (b430); exercise tolerance functions (b455)

Sources of information:
☒ Case history ☐ Patient-reported questionnaire ☒ Clinical examination ☒ Technical investigation

Description of the problem:
Complains of pain in the left lower leg when walking, pain disappears when resting; Ultrasonic pulsed Doppler analysis: Reduced blood circulation in the lower leg.

b420⁺	**Blood pressure functions**	0	1	**2**	3	4	8	9

Functions of maintaining the pressure of blood within the arteries.
Inclusions: functions of maintenance of blood pressure; increased and decreased blood pressure; impairments such as in hypotension, hypertension and postural hypotension
Exclusions: heart functions (b410); blood vessel functions (b415); exercise tolerance functions (b455)

Sources of information:
☒ Case history ☐ Patient-reported questionnaire ☒ Clinical examination ☐ Technical investigation

Description of the problem:
Blood pressure measure: 160/90 in rest, Hypertension.

b440	**Respiration functions**	**0**	1	2	3	4	8	9

Functions of inhaling air into the lungs, the exchange of gases between air and blood, and exhaling air.
Inclusions: functions of respiration rate, rhythm and depth; impairments such as apnoea, hyperventilation, irregular respiration, paradoxical respiration and bronchial spasm and as in pulmonary emphysema.
Exclusions: respiratory muscle functions (b445); additional respiratory functions (b450); exercise tolerance functions (b455)

Sources of information:
☒ Case history ☐ Patient-reported questionnaire ☒ Clinical examination ☐ Technical investigation

Description of the problem:
Respiration rate: 14/min, normal rhythm and movement, no secretion or other abnormalitly.

b455	**Exercise tolerance functions**	0	1	**2**	3	4	8	9

Functions of the muscles involved in breathing.
Inclusions: functions of thoracic respiratory muscles; functions of the diaphragm; functions of accessory respiratory muscles
Exclusions: respiration functions (b440); additional respiratory functions (b450); exercise tolerance functions (b455)

Sources of information:
☐ Case history ☐ Patient-reported questionnaire ☒ Clinical examination ☐ Technical investigation

Description of the problem:
Walking is exhaustive and increases heart rate and respiration rate after a short distance.

Figure 10. Continued on next page

b525	Defecation functions	**0**	1	2	3	4	8	9

Functions of elimination of wastes and undigested food as faeces and related functions.
Inclusions: functions of elimination, faecal consistency, frequency of defecation; faecal continence, flatulence; impairments such as constipation, diarrhoea, watery stool and anal sphincter incompetence or incontinence
Exclusions: digestive functions (b515); assimilation functions (b520); sensations associated with the digestive system (b535)

Sources of information:
☒ Case history ☐ Patient-reported questionnaire ☐ Clinical examination ☐ Technical investigation

Description of the problem: –

b620	Urination functions	**0**	1	2	3	4	8	9

Functions of discharge of urine from the urinary bladder.
Inclusions: functions of urination, frequency of urination, urinary continence; impairments such as in stress, urge, reflex, overflow, continuous incontinence, dribbling, automatic bladder, polyuria, urinary retention and urinary urgency
Exclusions: urinary excretory functions (b610); sensations associated with urinary functions (b630)

Sources of information:
☒ Case history ☐ Patient-reported questionnaire ☐ Clinical examination ☐ Technical investigation

Description of the problem: –

b710	Mobility of joint functions	0	**1**	2	3	4	8	9

Functions of the range and ease of movement of a joint.
Inclusions: functions of mobility of single or several joints, vertebral, shoulder, elbow, wrist, hip, knee, ankle, small joints of hands and feet; mobility of joints generalized; impairments such as in hypermobility of joints, frozen joints, frozen shoulder, arthritis
Exclusions: stability of joint functions (b715); control of voluntary movement functions (b760)

Sources of information:
☐ Case history ☐ Patient-reported questionnaire ☒ Clinical examination ☐ Technical investigation

Description of the problem:
Measurement of joint mobility with goniometer:

	left	*right*
Hip joint Abd-Add	*40 – 0 – 20*	*20 – 0 –20*
Hip joint Ext-Flex	*0 – 0 – 110*	*0 – 0 – 70*

b735	Exercise tolerance functions	0	1	**2**	3	4	8	9

Functions related to the tension present in the resting muscles and the resistance offered when trying to move the muscles passively.
Inclusions: functions associated with the tension of isolated muscles and muscle groups, muscles of one limb, one side of the body and the lower half of the body, muscles of all limbs, muscles of the trunk, and all muscles of the body; impairments such as hypotonia, hypertonia and muscle spasticity
Exclusions: muscle power functions (b730); muscle endurance functions (b740)

Sources of information:
☐ Case history ☐ Patient-reported questionnaire ☒ Clinical examination ☐ Technical investigation

Description of the problem:
Test of muscle elasticity: Increased muscle tone in Mm. adductors (right); Mm. ischiocrurale, Mm. adductors and M. triceps surae (left)

Figure 10. Continued on next page

BODY STRUCTURES
= anatomical parts of the body such as organs, limbs and their components

How much impairment does the person have in the...

Code	Category	Qualifier	No impairment	Mild impairment		Moderate impairment		Severe impairment		Complete impairment	Not specified	Not applicable
s410	**Structure of lower extremity**	Extent	0	1		2		**[3]**		4	8	9
		Nature*	0	1	2	3	4	5	6	**[7]**	8	9
		Location**	0	1	2	**[3]**	4	5	6	7	8	9

Sources of information:
☒ Case history ☐ Patient-reported questionnaire ☐ Clinical examination ☒ Technical investigation

Description of the problem:
Vascular impairments in the heart and lower legs. Artificial aortic and mitral valves.

Code	Category	Qualifier	No impairment	Mild impairment		Moderate impairment		Severe impairment		Complete impairment	Not specified	Not applicable
s710	**Structure of head and neck region**	Extent	**[0]**	1		2		3		4	8	9
		Nature*	0	1	2	3	4	5	6	7	8	9
		Location**	0	1	2	3	4	5	6	7	8	9

Sources of information:
☒ Case history ☐ Patient-reported questionnaire ☐ Clinical examination ☐ Technical investigation

Description of the problem: –

Code	Category	Qualifier	No impairment	Mild impairment		Moderate impairment		Severe impairment		Complete impairment	Not specified	Not applicable
s730	**Structure of upper extremity**	Extent	**[0]**	1		2		3		4	8	9
		Nature*	0	1	2	3	4	5	6	7	8	9
		Location**	0	1	2	3	4	5	6	7	8	9

Sources of information:
☒ Case history ☐ Patient-reported questionnaire ☐ Clinical examination ☐ Technical investigation

Description of the problem: –

Code	Category	Qualifier	No impairment	Mild impairment		Moderate impairment		Severe impairment		Complete impairment	Not specified	Not applicable
s740	**Structure of pelvic region**	Extent	**[0]**	1		2		3		4	8	9
		Nature*	0	1	2	3	4	5	6	7	8	9
		Location**	0	1	2	3	4	5	6	7	8	9

Sources of information:
☒ Case history ☐ Patient-reported questionnaire ☐ Clinical examination ☐ Technical investigation

Description of the problem: –

Code	Category	Qualifier	No impairment	Mild impairment		Moderate impairment		Severe impairment		Complete impairment	Not specified	Not applicable
s760	**Structure of trunk**	Extent	**[0]**	1		2		3		4	8	9
		Nature*	0	1	2	3	4	5	6	7	8	9
		Location**	0	1	2	3	4	5	6	7	8	9

Sources of information:
☒ Case history ☐ Patient-reported questionnaire ☐ Clinical examination ☐ Technical investigation

Description of the problem: –

Figure 10. Continued on next page

s810	Structure of areas of skin	Extent	0	1	**2**	3	4	8	9			
		Nature*	0	1	2	3	4	5	6	**7**	8	9
		Location**	0	**1**	2	3	4	5	6	7	8	9

Sources of information:

☐ Case history ☐ Patient-reported questionnaire ☒ Clinical examination ☐ Technical investigation

Description of the problem:

Inspection: Wound due to amputation not healed yet.

ACTIVITIES AND PARTICIPATION = execution of a task or action by an individual and involvement in a life situation *How much difficulty does the person have in the...* ***P** = performance of...* ***C** = capacity in...*			No difficulty	Mild difficulty	Moderate difficulty	Severe difficulty	Complete difficulty	Not specified	Not applicable
d230∞	**Carrying out daily routine**	P	**0**	1	2	3	4	8	9
		C	**0**	1	2	3	4	8	9

Carrying out simple or complex and coordinated actions in order to plan, manage and complete the requirements of day-to-day procedures or duties, such as budgeting time and making plans for separate activities throughout the day.
Inclusions: managing and completing the daily routine; managing one's own activity level
Exclusion: undertaking multiple tasks (d220)

Sources of information:

☒ Case history ☐ Patient-reported questionnaire ☐ Clinical examination ☐ Technical investigation

Description of the problem:

P: –
C: –

d240	Handling stress and other psychological demands	P	**0**	1	2	3	4	8	9
		C	**0**	1	2	3	4	8	9

Carrying out simple or complex and coordinated actions to manage and control the psychological demands required to carry out tasks demanding significant responsibilities and involving stress, distraction, or crises, such as driving a vehicle during heavy traffic or taking care of many children.
Inclusions: handling responsibilities; handling stress and crisis

Sources of information:

☒ Case history ☐ Patient-reported questionnaire ☐ Clinical examination ☐ Technical investigation

Description of the problem:

P: –
C: –

Figure 10. Continued on next page

d410	Changing basic body position								
		P	**0**	1	2	3	4	8	9
		C	0	1	2	**3**	4	8	9

Getting into and out of a body position and moving from one location to another, such as getting up out of a chair to lie down on a bed, and getting into and out of positions of kneeling or squatting.
Inclusions: changing body position from lying down, from squatting or kneeling, from sitting or standing, bending and shifting the body's centre of gravity
Exclusion: transferring oneself (d420)

Sources of information:
☐ Case history ☐ Patient-reported questionnaire ☒ Clinical examination ☐ Technical investigation

Description of the problem:
P: *With the walking frame no problem in changing the body position from sitting to standing.*
C: *To get into a standing position without an assistive device is quite instable and leads to an increased risk for falling. A walking frame is essential.*

d415	Maintaining a body position								
		P	**0**	1	2	3	4	8	9
		C	0	1	**2**	3	4	8	9

Staying in the same body position as required, such as remaining seated or remaining standing for work or school.
Inclusions: maintaining a lying, squatting, kneeling, sitting and standing position

Sources of information:
☐ Case history ☐ Patient-reported questionnaire ☒ Clinical examination ☐ Technical investigation

Description of the problem:
P: *With a walking frame no problems in standing*
C: *To maintain a standing position without devices is possible only for some seconds and severely instable. High risk for falling.*

d420	Transferring oneself								
		P	**0**	1	2	3	4	8	9
		C	**0**	1	2	3	4	8	9

Moving from one surface to another, such as sliding along a bench or moving from a bed to a chair, without changing body position.
Inclusion: transferring oneself while sitting or lying Exclusion: changing basic body position (d410)

Sources of information:
☐ Case history ☐ Patient-reported questionnaire ☒ Clinical examination ☐ Technical investigation

Description of the problem:
P: –
C: –

d450	Walking								
		P	0	1	2	**3**	4	8	9
		C	0	1	2	3	**4**	8	9

Moving along a surface on foot, step by step, so that one foot is always on the ground, such as when strolling, sauntering, walking forwards, backwards, or sideways.
Inclusions: walking short or long distances; walking on different surfaces; walking around obstacles
Exclusions: transferring oneself (d420); moving around (d455)

Sources of information:
☐ Case history ☐ Patient-reported questionnaire ☒ Clinical examination ☐ Technical investigation

Description of the problem:
P: *With devices, walking distance is severely reduced due to lack of muscle endurance in the upper body and left leg: with walking frame 50m, with crutches 15m.*
C: *Without devices walking is impossible.*

Figure 10. Continued on next page

d450∞	Moving around	P	0	1	2	3	**4**	8	9
		C	0	1	2	3	**4**	8	9

Moving the whole body from one place to another by means other than walking, such as climbing over a rock or running down a street, skipping, scampering, jumping, somersaulting or running around obstacles.
Inclusions: crawling, climbing, running, jogging, jumping, and swimming
Exclusions: transferring oneself (d420); walking (d450)

Sources of information:
☒ Case history ☐ Patient-reported questionnaire ☒ Clinical examination ☐ Technical investigation

Description of the problem:
P: *Is not able to move around in any other way than walking with devices.*
C: *Is not able to move around in any other way than walking with devices.*

d510	Washing oneself	P	**0**	1	2	3	4	8	9
		C	**0**	1	2	3	4	8	9

Washing and drying one's whole body, or body parts, using water and appropriate cleaning and drying materials or methods, such as bathing, showering, washing hands and feet, face and hair, and drying with a towel.
Inclusions: washing body parts, the whole body; and drying oneself
Exclusions: caring for body parts (d520); toileting (d530)

Sources of information:
☒ Case history ☐ Patient-reported questionnaire ☒ Clinical examination ☐ Technical investigation

Description of the problem:
P: –
C: –

d520	Caring for body parts	P	**0**	1	2	3	4	8	9
		C	**0**	1	2	3	4	8	9

Looking after those parts of the body, such as skin, face, teeth, scalp, nails and genitals, that requires more than washing and drying.
Inclusions: caring for skin, teeth, hair, finger and toe nails
Exclusions: washing oneself (d510); toileting (d530)

Sources of information:
☒ Case history ☐ Patient-reported questionnaire ☒ Clinical examination ☐ Technical investigation

Description of the problem:
P: –
C: –

d530	Toileting	P	**0**	1	2	3	4	8	9
		C	**0**	1	2	3	4	8	9

Planning and carrying out the elimination of human waste (menstruation, urination and defecation), and cleaning oneself afterwards.
Inclusions: regulating urination, defecation and menstrual care
Exclusions: washing oneself (d510); caring for body parts (d520)

Sources of information:
☒ Case history ☐ Patient-reported questionnaire ☐ Clinical examination ☐ Technical investigation

Description of the problem:
P: –
C: –

Figure 10. Continued on next page

d550	Eating	P	**0**	1	2	3	4	8	9
		C	**0**	1	2	3	4	8	9

Carrying out the coordinated tasks and actions of eating food that has been served, bringing it to the mouth and consuming it in culturally acceptable ways, cutting or breaking food into pieces, opening bottles and cans, using eating implements, having meals, feasting or dining.
Exclusion: drinking (d560)

Sources of information:
☒ Case history ☐ Patient-reported questionnaire ☐ Clinical examination ☐ Technical investigation

Description of the problem:
P: –
C: –

d850∞	Remunerative employment	P	0	1	2	3	4	8	**9**
		C	0	1	2	3	4	8	**9**

Engaging in all aspects of work, as an occupation, trade, profession or other form of employment, for payment, as an employee, full or part time, or self-employed, such as seeking employment and getting a job, doing the required tasks of the job, attending work on time as required, supervising other workers or being supervised, and performing required tasks alone or in groups.
Inclusions: self-employment, part-time and full-time employment

Sources of information:
☒ Case history ☐ Patient-reported questionnaire ☐ Clinical examination ☐ Technical investigation

Description of the problem:
P: *Patient is already retired.*
C: –

ENVIRONMENTAL FACTORS = make up the physical, social and attitudinal environment in which people live and conduct their lives. ***How much of a facilitator or barrier does the person experience with respect to...***		Complete facilitator	Substantial facilitator	Moderate facilitator	Mild facilitator	No barrier/facilitator	Mild barrier	Moderate barrier	Substantial barrier	Complete barrier	Not specified	Not applicable
e110	Products or substances for personal consumption	**+4**	+3	+2	+1	0	1	2	3	4	8	9

Any natural or human-made object or substance gathered, processed or manufactured for ingestion.
Inclusions: food, drink and drugs

Sources of information:
☒ Case history ☐ Patient-reported questionnaire ☒ Clinical examination ☒ Technical investigation

Description of the facilitator/barrier:
Receives medication, adapted to his condition: Ibuprofen, Novalgin, Diovam, Aspirin, Mono Embolex 8000

e355	Health professionals	**+4**	+3	+2	+1	0	1	2	3	4	8	9

All service providers working within the context of the health system, such as doctors, nurses, physiotherapists, occupational therapists, speech therapists, audiologists, orthotist-prosthetists, medical social workers.
Exclusion: other professionals (e360)

Sources of information:
☒ Case history ☐ Patient-reported questionnaire ☐ Clinical examination ☐ Technical investigation

Description of the facilitator/barrier:
Receives support from medical doctor, nurse, physical therapist, orthopedic technician and social worker

Figure 10. Continued on next page

e420	Individual attitudes of friends	+4	+3	+2	+1	0	1	2	3	4	8	9
	General or specific opinions and beliefs of friends about the person or about other matters (e.g. social, political and economic issues), that influence individual behaviour and actions.											
	Sources of information: ☒ Case history ☐ Patient-reported questionnaire ☐ Clinical examination ☐ Technical investigation											
	Description of the facilitator/barrier: *Friends are very positive and willing to support him whenever required*											

Figure 10
Documentation form based on the ICF Core Set for Musculoskeletal Conditions in Acute Care (Brief version)

Note. ICF categories marked in dark grey belong to the Generic Set and are included in any documentation form

∞ Category from the Generic Set not included in the ICF Core Set for Musculoskeletal Conditions in Acute Care

+ Category selected from the ICF Core Set for Chronic Ischaemic Heart Disease

* Rating of the nature of the impairment in Body Structures: 0 = no change in structure, 1 = total absence, 2 = partial absence, 3 = additional part, 4 = aberrant dimension, 5 = discontinuity, 6 = deviating position, 7 = qualitative changes in structure, 8 = not specified, 9 = not applicable

** Rating of the location of the impairment in Body Structures: 0 = more than one region, 1 = right, 2 = left, 3 = both sides, 4 = front, 5 = back, 6 = proximal, 7 = distal, 8 = not specified, 9 = not applicable

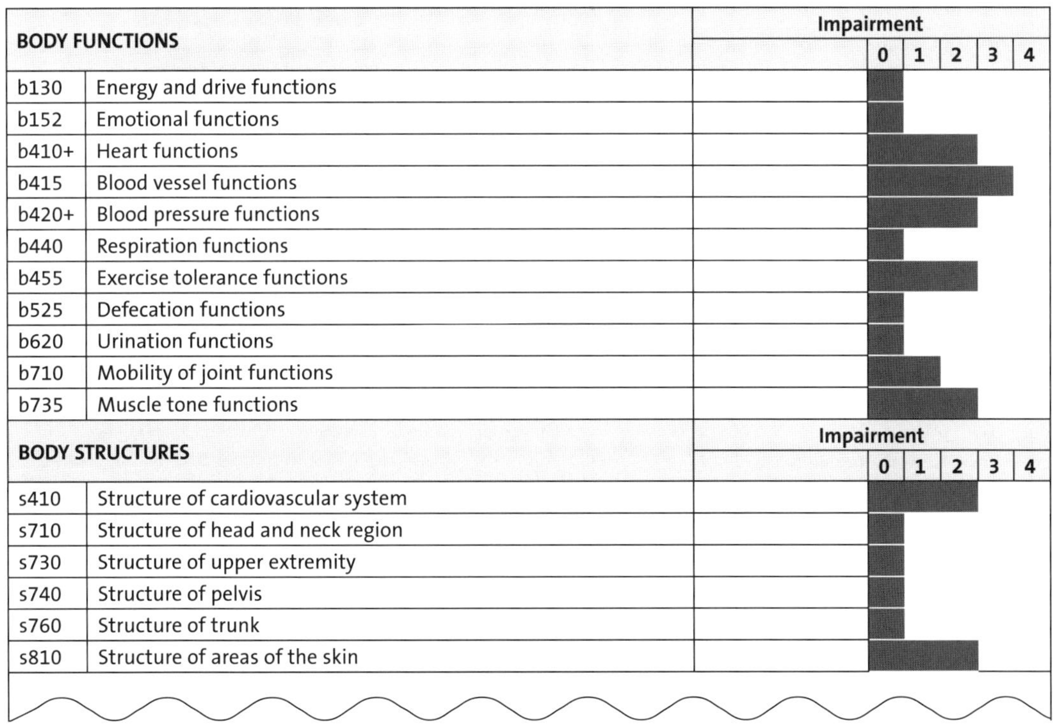

BODY FUNCTIONS			Impairment				
			0	1	2	3	4
b130	Energy and drive functions						
b152	Emotional functions						
b410+	Heart functions						
b415	Blood vessel functions						
b420+	Blood pressure functions						
b440	Respiration functions						
b455	Exercise tolerance functions						
b525	Defecation functions						
b620	Urination functions						
b710	Mobility of joint functions						
b735	Muscle tone functions						
BODY STRUCTURES			**Impairment**				
			0	1	2	3	4
s410	Structure of cardiovascular system						
s710	Structure of head and neck region						
s730	Structure of upper extremity						
s740	Structure of pelvis						
s760	Structure of trunk						
s810	Structure of areas of the skin						

Figure 11. Continued on next page

ACTIVITIES AND PARTICIPATION			Difficulty 0 1 2 3 4
d230∞	Carrying out daily routine	P	
		C	
d240	Handling stress and other psychological demands	P	
		C	
d410	Changing basic body position	P	
		C	
d415	Maintaining a body position	P	
		C	
d420	Transferring oneself	P	
		C	
d450	Walking	P	
		C	
d455∞	Moving around	P	
		C	
d510	Washing oneself	P	
		C	
d520	Caring for body parts	P	
		C	
d530	Toileting	P	
		C	
d550	Eating	P	
		C	
d850∞	Remunerative employment	P	9
		C	

ENVIRONMENTAL FACTORS		Facilitator +4 +3 +2 +1 0	Barrier 1 2 3 4
e110	Products or substances for personal consumption		
e115	Products and technology for personal use in daily living		
e120	Products and techn. for pers. indoor and outdoor mobility and transportation		
e310	Immediate family		
e320	Friends		
e355	Health professionals		
e410	Individual attitudes of immediate family members		
e420	Individual attitudes of friends		
e455	Individual attitudes of health-related professionals		
e580	Health services, systems and policies		

Figure 11

Functioning profile of a person with a musculoskeletal condition (amputation) in acute care (Brief version)

Note. In Body Functions, Body Structures, Activities and Participation: 0 = no problem, 1 = mild problem, 2 = moderate problem, 3 = severe problem, 4 = complete problem; In Environmental Factors: 0 = no barrier/facilitator, 1 = mild barrier, 2 = moderate barrier, 3=severe barrier, 4 = complete barrier, +1 = mild facilitator, +2 = moderate facilitator, +3 = substantial facilitator, +4 = complete facilitator, 8 = not specified, 9 = not applicable

P = Performance, C = Capacity

∞ ICF categories from the Generic Set not included in the ICF Core Set for Musculoskeletal Conditions in Acute Care

+ ICF categories added to the ICF Core Set for Musculoskeletal Conditions in Acute Care

5.1.6. Discussion – Applying ICF Core Sets to Persons with Several Health Conditions

The selection of the appropriate ICF Core Set is based on the person's existing diagnosis and the health service context (acute, post-acute or long term) in which the description of functioning will be used. Usually, the health service context in which a patient finds him- or herself determines whether an ICF Core Set for a health condition or an ICF Core Set for a condition group – which includes several specific health conditions – will be selected. Selecting the appropriate ICF Core Set is an easy task when a person suffers from only one health condition. What is required when a patient has multiple health conditions? In such cases, there are a couple of options:

- choose only one ICF Core Set for the main diagnosis for which treatment is planned
- choose one ICF Core Set for the main diagnosis for which treatment is planned and add appropriate ICF categories from other ICF Core Sets or from the whole ICF
- combine all ICF categories from ICF Core Sets related to the health conditions or condition groups that are relevant to the patient

In this use case, Mr. Miller was admitted to an acute health service for the amputation of his right leg, although he suffered from five other underlying diseases: peripheral arterial obstructive disease (ICD: "I73.9 Peripheral vascular disease, unspecified"); thrombosis in the right leg (ICD: "I74.3 Arterial embolism and thrombosis of lower extremities"); diabetes mellitus (ICD: "E10 Insulin-dependent diabetes mellitus"); arterial hypertension (ICD: "I10 Essential primary hypertension"); insufficiency of (artificial) mitral and aortic valves (ICD 10: "I34.0 Mitral valve insufficiency" and "I35.1 Aortic valve insufficiency"). Most of these diseases are vascular in nature. The thrombosis in the right leg needed treatment and was the reason for the patient's hospital admission. The consequential right femoral amputation led to the current and acute problems in functioning. To address all of the health issues in this case, the ICF Core Set for Musculoskeletal Conditions in Acute Care is most appropriate, since it includes amputation. The ICF Core Sets for Cardiopulmonary Conditions or the ICF Core Set for Diabetes Mellitus – although they address many of Mr. Miller's potential problems in functioning related to his existing cardiovascular diseases – were not selected because neither would address his actual and current primary problems in functioning, all of which are related to the amputation. To take into account the patient's cardiovascular diseases in more detail, however, two additional ICF categories describing *heart functions (b410)* and *blood pressure functions (b420)* were selected from the ICF Core Set for

Cardiopulmonary Conditions in Acute Care since they were viewed to be important in this case.

This use case illustrates the process of selecting an ICF Core Set for a person with multiple health conditions in the acute phase. It shows the need for clinical judgment and an awareness of the specific details of the case. Adding ICF categories from other ICF Core Sets or combining different ICF Core Sets allows users to create a list of ICF categories that are best suited to the specific details and patterns of functioning problems experienced by the individual patient.

5.2. Use Case 2: Applying the Comprehensive ICF Core Set for Spinal Cord Injury in Post-Acute Care

Alexandra Rauch

This use case illustrates the application of an ICF Core Set to a patient who suffers from spinal cord injury (SCI) as a result of a traffic accident and who is currently undergoing rehabilitation in a specialized SCI rehabilitation centre. The case also discusses the implementation of ICF Core Sets in multidisciplinary settings.

5.2.1. The Case

Mr. Smith, a 26-year-old man, sustained a SCI (ICD: S24) as a result of a fractured 7th and 8th thoracic vertebrae in a motorcycle accident. In the accident, Mr. Smith also suffered a lung contusion and a strained left knee. Emergency spinal surgery was performed on the same day of the accident to stabilize the fractures of the spine. The procedure required movement restriction of the spine (no rotation, no flexion) for three months to ensure healing of the fracture. Despite optimal acute care, he had complete loss of motor and sensory function below the lesion level (7th thoracic vertebra).

Before the accident, Mr. Smith worked as a mover, although he was trained as a salesman for consumer electronics. He was single, but shared a wheelchair inaccessible apartment with a good friend. He spent his free time riding his motor bike, playing golf and socializing with his friends and family.

Two days after the surgery, Mr. Smith was admitted to a centre specialized in SCI rehabilitation. He was directly admitted to the post-acute rehabilitation unit of the centre. In this unit, a comprehensive rehabilitation program was started. From the beginning, Mr. Smith's level of functioning steadily improved, however, the recovery was not as fast as he had wished, due to the movement restrictions by the surgeon. Three months later, the restrictions could be removed and Mr. Smith could be prepared for discharge home. At this time-point, the comprehensive rehabilitation program should be intensified and all requirements for successful community integration should be integrated into the rehabilitation management.

5.2.2. The Application Area and Setting

The rehabilitation centre is located in Switzerland and specializes in treatment within acute, post-acute and long-term care of SCI and includes inpatient (for acute, post-acute and long-term care) and outpatient services (only for long-term care). In order to implement a comprehensive rehabilitation strategy, the rehabilitation management team needs to address all of the needs associated with the problems related to his SCI. These include medical care and nursing, physical, occupational, sports and psychological therapy, vocational rehabilitation, social worker's support to clarify financial issues related to housing, motorization, provision of assistive devices, adaptation of housing and so on. Because of these needs, the rehabilitation team is composed of several disciplines working together to achieve and maintain optimal functioning in all phases of SCI. The most important outcome of the post-acute rehabilitation program is to achieve successful community re-integration.

5.2.3. The Purpose of Applying the ICF Core Set

In this use case, the current rehabilitation cycle was initiated with a new assessment that served as the basis for the definition of rehabilitation goals, identification of intervention targets and the implementation and evaluation of interventions to achieve successful community re-integration. Complete information about Mr. Smith's level of functioning is therefore needed for rehabilitation planning. Whichever ICF Core Set is used, a comprehensive description of functioning is gained by integrating all areas of functioning and the environment, which then enables the team to help the patient to achieve the best possible physical and psychological functioning. The ICF Core Set must also provide a common language for several health professionals to share all available information about the patient's level of functioning.

5.2.4. Selection of the Appropriate ICF Core Set

The selection of the appropriate ICF Core Set was performed according to the health care context and the type of ICF Core Set (Figure 12).

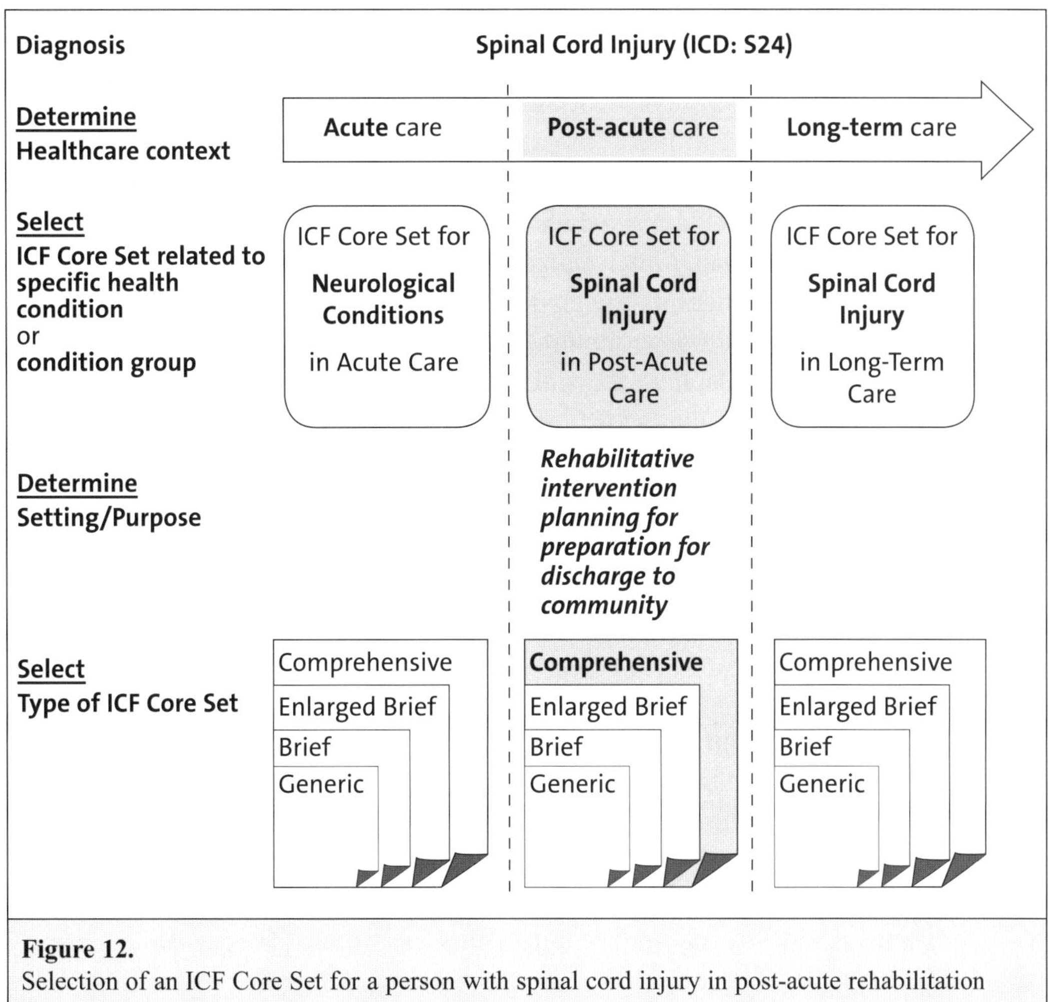

Figure 12.
Selection of an ICF Core Set for a person with spinal cord injury in post-acute rehabilitation

Choice of ICF Core Set Related to Specific Health Condition or Condition Group

To describe Mr. Smith's level of functioning, the *ICF Core Set for Spinal Cord Injury* was selected. For SCI, health condition-specific ICF Core Sets are available for both post-acute[33] and long-term care.[34] SCI is the only health condition for which a health condition-specific Core Set for application in the early post-acute setting exists. In this use case, the *ICF Core Set for Spinal Cord Injury in* ***Post-Acute Care*** was selected instead of the condition group *ICF Core Set for Neurological Conditions in Post-Acute Care.*[29]

ICF Core Sets for post-acute care cover the early part of rehabilitation when patients have both medical needs requiring hospital care and initial comprehensive rehabilitation directly after an acute illness or injury.[10] These ICF Core Sets have therefore been developed for use by physicians, nurses, therapists, other health professionals and other professionals working in the field of health care in rehabilitation programs.[28] Such programs are provided after the initial acute care and aim to restore and maintain functioning, to promote patient's autonomy and to prevent the need for long-term care by targeted interventions.[75] In addition, community integration is the main goal of rehabilitation, which depends not only on a person's physical functioning, but also on many interrelated facilitators and barriers in the social and physical environment. Rehabilitation teams therefore need to consider issues such as employment, mobility and transportation, family support and physical accessibility in the community when planning transition into the community.[34]

The *ICF Core Set for Spinal Cord Injury in Post-Acute Care* was developed for both traumatic and non-traumatic SCIs. The Comprehensive ICF Core Set includes a total of 162 2nd-, 3rd- or 4th-level categories and the brief version includes 25 2nd-level ICF categories.

Choice of the Type of ICF Core Set

For this case, the **Comprehensive** ICF Core Set was selected. Although this Comprehensive ICF Core Set consists of many categories, the selection of this type of Core Set ensures that no domain of functioning and the person's environment are overlooked as potential intervention targets. As noted, it is recommended that all of the ICF categories in the Generic Set not already included in a Comprehensive ICF Core Set should also be added, but in this case these categories are already included in the Comprehensive ICF Core Set for SCI, although the category *b280 Sensation of pain* of the Generic Set is presented by 3rd- and 4th-level categories in the Comprehensive ICF Core Set.

5.2.5. The Description of Functioning with the Documentation Form

For each ICF category, information was derived from a variety of sources: Mr. Smith's history, a clinical examination and technical investigations. For some areas of functioning, information was available from more than one source. In this use case, no patient-reported questionnaire was used. The information was gathered from team members and then rated by one team member using the ICF qualifiers. The following figures present the Brief version of the documentation form (Figure 13) and the functioning profile (consisting of all ICF categories from the Brief ICF Core Set for SCI in Post-Acute Care combined with the Generic Set; Figure 14). The full version is available on the CD included with this Manual.

<table>
<tr><td colspan="2">BODY FUNCTIONS
= physiological functions of body systems (including psychological functions)
How much of a problem does the person have in...</td><td>No problem</td><td>Mild problem</td><td>Moderate problem</td><td>Severe problem</td><td>Complete problem</td><td>Not specified</td><td>Not applicable</td></tr>
<tr><td>b130</td><td>Energy and drive functions</td><td>[0]</td><td>1</td><td>2</td><td>3</td><td>4</td><td>8</td><td>9</td></tr>
<tr><td></td><td colspan="8">General mental functions of physiological and psychological mechanisms that cause the individual to move towards satisfying specific needs and general goals in a persistent manner.
Inclusions: functions of energy level, motivation, appetite, craving (including craving for substances that can be abused), and impulse control
Exclusions: consciousness functions (b110); temperament and personality functions (b126); sleep functions (b134); psychomotor functions (b147); emotional functions (b152)</td></tr>
<tr><td></td><td colspan="8">Sources of information:
☒ Case history ☐ Patient-reported questionnaire ☐ Clinical examination ☐ Technical investigation</td></tr>
<tr><td></td><td colspan="8">Description of the problem:
Very motivated to work on the improvements of his Functioning level – presents a good resource</td></tr>
<tr><td>b152</td><td>Emotional functions</td><td>[0]</td><td>1</td><td>2</td><td>3</td><td>4</td><td>8</td><td>9</td></tr>
<tr><td></td><td colspan="8">Specific mental functions related to the feeling and affective components of the processes of the mind.
Inclusions: functions of appropriateness of emotion, regulation and range of emotion; affect; sadness, happiness, love, fear, anger, hate, tension, anxiety, joy, sorrow; lability of emotion; flattening of affect
Exclusions: temperament and personality functions (b126); energy and drive functions (b130)</td></tr>
<tr><td></td><td colspan="8">Sources of information:
☒ Case history ☐ Patient-reported questionnaire ☐ Clinical examination ☐ Technical investigation</td></tr>
<tr><td></td><td colspan="8">Description of the problem:
Emotional functions appropriate to actual situation</td></tr>
<tr><td>b280</td><td>Sensation of pain</td><td>0</td><td>[1]</td><td>2</td><td>3</td><td>4</td><td>8</td><td>9</td></tr>
<tr><td></td><td colspan="8">Sensation of unpleasant feeling indicating potential or actual damage to some body structure felt all over or throughout the body.</td></tr>
<tr><td></td><td colspan="8">Sources of information:
☒ Case history ☐ Patient-reported questionnaire ☒ Clinical examination ☐ Technical investigation</td></tr>
<tr><td></td><td colspan="8">Description of the problem:
Slight neuropathic pain when moving the legs. Rated on Visual Analog Scale (0–10) as 2</td></tr>
<tr><td>b440</td><td>Respiration functions</td><td>[0]</td><td>1</td><td>2</td><td>3</td><td>4</td><td>8</td><td>9</td></tr>
<tr><td></td><td colspan="8">Functions of inhaling air into the lungs, the exchange of gases between air and blood, and exhaling air.
Inclusions: functions of respiration rate, rhythm and depth; impairments such as apnoea, hyperventilation, irregular respiration, paradoxical respiration and bronchial spasm and as in pulmonary emphysema.
Exclusions: respiratory muscle functions (b445); additional respiratory functions (b450); exercise tolerance functions (b455)</td></tr>
<tr><td></td><td colspan="8">Sources of information:
☐ Case history ☐ Patient-reported questionnaire ☒ Clinical examination ☐ Technical investigation</td></tr>
<tr><td></td><td colspan="8">Description of the problem:
Measurement of breathing rhythm and rate per minute: regular rhythm and rate; no subjective problems reported by patient. Spinal Cord Idependence Measure (SCIM)-Respiration: 10 (= Breathes independently without assistance or devices)</td></tr>
</table>

Figure 13. Continued on next page

Code	Category	0	1	2	3	4	8	9
b525	Defecation functions	0	1	2	3	**4**	8	9

Consistency of faeces such as hard, firm, soft or watery.

Sources of information:

☒ Case history ☐ Patient-reported questionnaire ☒ Clinical examination ☐ Technical investigation

Description of the problem:

Due to loss of voluntary control faecal incontinence

Code	Category	0	1	2	3	4	8	9
b620	Urination functions	0	1	2	3	**4**	8	9

Functions of voiding the urinary bladder.
Inclusions: impairments such as in urine retention

Sources of information:

☒ Case history ☐ Patient-reported questionnaire ☒ Clinical examination ☐ Technical investigation

Description of the problem:

Complete incontinence due to loss of voluntary control. requires intermittent catheterization

Code	Category	0	1	2	3	4	8	9
b730	Muscle power functions	0	1	2	3	**4**	8	9

Functions related to the force generated by the contraction of specific and isolated muscles and muscle groups.
Inclusion: impairments such as weakness of small muscles of feet or hands

Sources of information:

☐ Case history ☐ Patient-reported questionnaire ☒ Clinical examination ☐ Technical investigation

Description of the problem:

Manual muscle testing (MMT) resulted in 0 (total paralysis) in all muscles below the level of injury

Code	Category	0	1	2	3	4	8	9
b735	Muscle tone functions	0	1	**2**	3	4	8	9

Functions related to the tension present in the resting muscles and muscle groups in the lower half of the body and the resistance offered when trying to move those muscles passively.
Inclusions: impairments associated with paraparesis and paraplegia

Sources of information:

☐ Case history ☐ Patient-reported questionnaire ☒ Clinical examination ☐ Technical investigation

Description of the problem:

Increased muscle tone in the lower half of the body, associated with movement

Code	Category	0	1	2	3	4	8	9
b810	Protective functions of the skin	**0**	1	2	3	4	8	9

Functions of the skin for protecting the body from physical, chemical and biological threats.
Inclusions: functions of protecting against the sun and other radiation, photosensitivity, pigmentation, quality of skin; insulating function of skin, callus formation, hardening; impairments such as broken skin, ulcers, bedsores and thinning of skin
Exclusions: repair functions of the skin (b820); other functions of the skin (b830)

Sources of information:

☐ Case history ☐ Patient-reported questionnaire ☒ Clinical examination ☐ Technical investigation

Description of the problem:

Visual inspection: No existing pressure sores

Figure 13. Continued on next page

BODY STRUCTURES = anatomical parts of the body such as organs, limbs and their components ***How much impairment does the person have in the...***			No impairment	Mild impairment	Moderate impairment	Severe impairment	Complete impairment	Not specified	Not applicable
s120	Spinal cord and related structures	Extent	0	1	2	3	**4**	8	9
		Nature*	0	1 2 3 4 **5** 6 7				8	9
		Location**	0	1 2 3 4 5 **6** 7				8	9

Sources of information:

☐ Case history ☐ Patient-reported questionnaire ☒ Clinical examination ☒ Technical investigation

Description of the problem:

MRI, Asia Impairment Score (AIS): Complete impairment of the spinal cord at 7th thoracic vertebra

s430	Structure of respiratory system	Extent	**0**	1	2	3	4	8	9
		Nature*	0	1 2 3 4 5 6 7				8	9
		Location**	0	1 2 3 4 5 6 7				8	9

Sources of information:

☒ Case history ☐ Patient-reported questionnaire ☐ Clinical examination ☐ Technical investigation

Description of the problem: –

s610	Structure of urinary system	Extent	**0**	1	2	3	4	8	9
		Nature*	0	1 2 3 4 5 6 7				8	9
		Location**	0	1 2 3 4 5 6 7				8	9

Sources of information:

☒ Case history ☐ Patient-reported questionnaire ☐ Clinical examination ☐ Technical investigation

Description of the problem:

No changes found through ultrasound

ACTIVITIES AND PARTICIPATION = execution of a task or action by an individual and involvement in a life situation ***How much of a problem does the person have in the...*** ***P = performance of...*** ***C = capacity in...***			No problem	Mild problem	Moderate problem	Severe problem	Complete problem	Not specified	Not applicable
d230	Carrying out daily routine	P	**0**	1	2	3	4	8	9
		C	**0**	1	2	3	4	8	9

Carrying out simple or complex and coordinated actions in order to plan, manage and complete the requirements of day-to-day procedures or duties, such as budgeting time and making plans for separate activities throughout the day.
Inclusions: managing and completing the daily routine; managing one's own activity level
Exclusion: undertaking multiple tasks (d220)

Sources of information:

☒ Case history ☐ Patient-reported questionnaire ☐ Clinical examination ☐ Technical investigation

Description of the problem:

P: *No difficulty*
C: *No difficulty*

Figure 13. Continued on next page

d360	Using communication devices and techniques								
		P	**0**	1	2	3	4	8	9
		C	**0**	1	2	3	4	8	9

Using devices, techniques and other means for the purposes of communicating, such as calling a friend on the telephone.
Inclusions: handling responsibilities; handling stress and crisis

Sources of information:

☒ Case history ☐ Patient-reported questionnaire ☐ Clinical examination ☐ Technical investigation

Description of the problem:

P: *No difficulty*
C: *No difficulty*

d410	Changing basic body position								
		P	0	1	**2**	3	4	8	9
		C	0	1	2	3	**4**	8	9

Getting into and out of a body position and moving from one location to another, such as getting up out of a chair to lie down on a bed, and getting into and out of positions of kneeling or squatting.
Inclusions: changing body position from lying down, from squatting or kneeling, from sitting or standing, bending and shifting the body's centre of gravity
Exclusion: transferring oneself (d420)

Sources of information:

☐ Case history ☐ Patient-reported questionnaire ☒ Clinical examination ☐ Technical investigation

Description of the problem:

P: *With assistance in sitting up from lying position able to change body position slowly and carefully*
C: *Without assistance not able (not allowed) to sit up and lay down (due to restrictions related to spinal surgery, problems with shifting the body while sitting due to impaired muscle power and proprioceptive functions*

d420	Transferring oneself								
		P	0	**1**	2	3	4	8	9
		C	0	1	**2**	3	4	8	9

Moving from one surface to another, such as sliding along a bench or moving from a bed to a chair, without changing body position.
Inclusion: transferring oneself while sitting or lying; Exclusion: changing basic body position (d410)

Sources of information:

☒ Case history ☐ Patient-reported questionnaire ☒ Clinical examination ☐ Technical investigation

Description of the problem:

P: *With the use of devices independent but increased time consumption*
C: *Requires a sliding board to transfer from bed to wheelchair and back, or to transfer into the car. SCIM-Transfer: 1 (= Needs partial assistance and/or supervision, and/or adaptive devices). Without devices some difficulties and increased risk for falls*

d450	Walking								
		P	0	1	2	3	**4**	8	9
		C	0	1	2	3	**4**	8	9

Walking for less than a kilometer, such as walking around rooms or hallways, within a building or for short distances outside.

Sources of information:

☒ Case history ☐ Patient-reported questionnaire ☐ Clinical examination ☐ Technical investigation

Description of the problem:

P: *Not able to walk at all*
C: *Not able to walk at all*

Figure 13. Continued on next page

Code	Category		0	1	2	3	4	8	9
d455	Moving around	P	0	1	2	3	**4**	8	9
		C	0	1	2	3	**4**	8	9

Moving the whole body from one place to another by means other than walking, such as climbing over a rock or running down a street, skipping, scampering, jumping, somersaulting or running around obstacles.
Inclusions: crawling, climbing, running, jogging, jumping, and swimming
Exclusions: transferring oneself (d420); walking (d450)

Sources of information:
☒ Case history ☐ Patient-reported questionnaire ☒ Clinical examination ☐ Technical investigation

Description of the problem:
P: *Not able to move in any other mean than moving the wheelchair*
C: *Not able to move around*

Code	Category		0	1	2	3	4	8	9
d510	Washing oneself	P	**0**	1	2	3	4	8	9
		C	0	**1**	2	3	4	8	9

Washing and drying one's whole body, or body parts, using water and appropriate cleaning and drying materials or methods, such as bathing, showering, washing hands and feet, face and hair, and drying with a towel.
Inclusions: washing body parts, the whole body; and drying oneself
Exclusions: caring for body parts (d520); toileting (d530)

Sources of information:
☒ Case history ☐ Patient-reported questionnaire ☒ Clinical examination ☐ Technical investigation

Description of the problem:
P: *Independent when using devices*
C: *Requires some little adaptations (handholds, shower wheelchair). SCIM-Bathing: 2 (= washes independently with adaptive devices or in a specific setting), without devices increased time consumption*

Code	Category		0	1	2	3	4	8	9
d530	Toileting	P	0	1	**2**	3	4	8	9
		C	0	1	2	3	**4**	8	9

Coordinating and managing urination, such as by indicating need, getting into the proper position, choosing and getting to an appropriate place for urination, manipulating clothing before and after urination, and cleaning oneself after urination

Sources of information:
☒ Case history ☐ Patient-reported questionnaire ☒ Clinical examination ☐ Technical investigation

Description of the problem:
P: *With devices independent in regulating urination but requires assistance for regulating defecation*
C: *Without devices completely limited. Using catheters and devices completely independent; SCIM-Sphincter management bladder: 11 (= Intermittent self-catheterization: continent between catheterizations; does not use external drainage instrument)*

Figure 13. Continued on next page

d540	Dressing								
		P	0	**1**	2	3	4	8	9
		C	0	1	**2**	3	4	8	9

Carrying out the coordinated actions and tasks of putting on and taking off clothes and footwear in sequence and in keeping with climatic and social conditions, such as by putting on, adjusting and removing shirts, skirts, blouses, pants, undergarments, saris, kimono, tights, hats, gloves, coats, shoes, boots, sandals and slippers.
Inclusions: putting on or taking off clothes and footwear and choosing appropriate clothing

Sources of information:

☒ Case history ☐ Patient-reported questionnaire ☒ Clinical examination ☐ Technical investigation

Description of the problem:

P: *With assistance still increased time consumption for dressing the lower body*
C: *Independent with dressing the upper body: SCIM-Dressing A: 4 (= Dresses any clothes independently; does not require adaptive devices or specific setting), needs partial assistance with dressing the lower body, SCIM-Dressing B:1 (= Requires partial assistance with clothes without buttons, zippers or laces)*

d550	Eating								
		P	**0**	1	2	3	4	8	9
		C	**0**	1	2	3	4	8	9

Carrying out the coordinated tasks and actions of eating food that has been served, bringing it to the mouth and consuming it in culturally acceptable ways, cutting or breaking food into pieces, opening bottles and cans, using eating implements, having meals, feasting or dining.
Exclusion: drinking (d560)

Sources of information:

☒ Case history ☐ Patient-reported questionnaire ☒ Clinical examination ☐ Technical investigation

Description of the problem:

P: *No difficulty*
C: *SCIM-Feeding: 3 (= Eats and drinks independently; does not require assistance or adaptive devices)*

d560	Drinking								
		P	**0**	1	2	3	4	8	9
		C	**0**	1	2	3	4	8	9

Taking hold of a drink, bringing it to the mouth and consuming the drink in culturally acceptable ways, mixing, stirring and pouring liquids for drinking, opening bottles and cans, drinking through a straw or drinking running water such as from a tap or a spring; feeding from the breast.
Exclusion: eating (d550)

Sources of information:

☒ Case history ☐ Patient-reported questionnaire ☒ Clinical examination ☐ Technical investigation

Description of the problem:

P: *No difficulty*
C: *SCIM-Feeding: 3 (= Eats and drinks independently; does not require assistance or adaptive devices)*

Figure 13. Continued on next page

d850	Remunerative employment	P	0	1	2	3	4	8	**9**
		C	0	1	2	3	**4**	8	9

Engaging in all aspects of work, as an occupation, trade, profession or other form of employment, for payment, as an employee, full or part time, or self-employed, such as seeking employment and getting a job, doing the required tasks of the job, attending work on time as required, supervising other workers or being supervised, and performing required tasks alone or in groups.
Inclusions: self-employment, part-time and full-time employment

Sources of information:
☒ Case history ☐ Patient-reported questionnaire ☐ Clinical examination ☐ Technical investigation

Description of the problem:
P: *Still at in-patient rehabilitation setting*
C: *Not able to work at the moment. Will not be able to work as a mover anymore but would be able to work part-time in a job that only requires sitting. No vocational solution found so far*

ENVIRONMENTAL FACTORS
= make up the physical, social and attitudinal environment in which people live and conduct their lives

How much of a facilitator or barrier does the person experience with respect to...

		Complete facilitator	Substantial facilitator	Moderate facilitator	Mild facilitator	No barrier/facilitator	Mild barrier	Moderate barrier	Severe barrier	Complete barrier	Not specified	Not applicable
e115	Products and technology for personal use in daily living	**+4**	+3	+2	+1	0	1	2	3	4	8	9
e120	Products and technology for personal indoor and outdoor mobility and transportation	+4	**+3**	+2	+1	0	1	2	3	4	8	9

e115

Equipment, products and technologies used by people in daily activities, including those adapted or specially designed, located in, on or near the person using them.
Inclusions: general and assistive products and technology for personal use

Sources of information:
☒ Case history ☐ Patient-reported questionnaire ☒ Clinical examination ☒ Technical investigation

Description of the facilitator/barrier:
Received various assistive devices and materials necessary for self-care and mobility that support him totally

e120

Equipment, products and technologies used by people in activities of moving inside and outside buildings, including those adapted or specially designed, located in, on or near the person using them
Inclusions: general and assistive products and technology for personal indoor and outdoor mobility and transportation

Sources of information:
☒ Case history ☐ Patient-reported questionnaire ☐ Clinical examination ☐ Technical investigation

Description of the facilitator/barrier:
Has manual wheelchair which is not completely adapted to his needs, will receive a motorized pulling machine for the wheelchair, car has to be adapted

Figure 13. Continued on next page

e310	Immediate family	**+4**	+3	+2	+1	0	1	2	3	4	8	9
	Individuals related by birth, marriage or other relationship recognized by the culture as immediate family, such as spouses, partners, parents, siblings, children, foster parents, adoptive parents and grandparents. *Exclusions: extended family (e315); personal care providers and personal assistants (e340)*											
	Sources of information: ☒ Case history ☐ Patient-reported questionnaire ☐ Clinical examination ☐ Technical investigation											
	Description of the facilitator/barrier: *Receives very much support from his family*											

e340	Personal care providers and personal assistants	+4	+3	+2	+1	0	1	2	3	4	8	**9**
	Individuals who provide services as required to support individuals in their daily activities and maintenance of performance at work, education ,or other life situation, provided either through public or private funds or else on a voluntary basis, such as providers of support for home-making and maintenance, personal assistants, transport assistants, paid help, nannies and others who function as primary caregivers. *Exclusions: immediate family (e310); extended family (e315); friends (e320); general social support services (e5750); health professionals (e355)*											
	Sources of information: ☒ Case history ☐ Patient-reported questionnaire ☐ Clinical examination ☐ Technical investigation											
	Description of the facilitator/barrier: *He has no specific personal care providers*											

e355	Health professionals	**+4**	+3	+2	+1	0	1	2	3	4	8	9
	All service providers working within the context of the health system, such as doctors, nurses, physiotherapists, occupational therapists, speech therapists, audiologists, orthotist-prosthetists, medical social workers. *Exclusion: other professionals (e360)*											
	Sources of information: ☒ Case history ☐ Patient-reported questionnaire ☐ Clinical examination ☐ Technical investigation											
	Description of the facilitator/barrier: *Health professionals are experienced as extremely supportive by the patient*											

Figure 13.
ICF Core Set based documentation form based on the ICF Core Set for Spinal Cord Injury in Post-Acute Care (Brief version)

ICF categories marked in dark grey belong to the Generic Set and are included in any documentation form

*Rating of the nature of the impairment in Body Structures: 0 = no change in structure, 1 = total absence, 2 = partial absence, 3 = additional part, 4 = aberrant dimension, 5 = discontinuity, 6 = deviating position, 7 = qualitative changes in structure, 8 = not specified, 9 = not applicable

** Rating of the location of the impairment in Body Structures: 0 = more than one region, 1 = right, 2 = left, 3 = both sides, 4 = front, 5 = back, 6 = proximal, 7 = distal, 8 = not specified, 9 = not applicable

BODY FUNCTIONS		**Impairment**				
		0	**1**	**2**	**3**	**4**
b130	Energy and drive functions					
b152	Emotional functions					
b270	Sensory functions related to temperature and other stimuli					
b280	Sensation of pain					
b440	Respiration functions					
b525	Defecation functions					
b620	Urination functions					
b730	Muscle power functions					
b735	Muscle tone functions					
b810	Protective functions of the skin					

BODY STRUCTURES		**Impairment**				
		0	**1**	**2**	**3**	**4**
s120	Spinal cord and related structures					
s430	Structure of respiratory system					
s610	Structure of urinary system					

ACTIVITIES AND PARTICIPATION			**Difficulty**				
			0	**1**	**2**	**3**	**4**
d230	Carrying out daily routine	P					
		C					
d410	Changing basic body positions	P					
		C					
d420	Transferring oneself	P					
		C					
d445	Hand and arm use	P					
		C					
d450	Walking	P					
		C					
d455	Moving around	P					
		C					
d510	Washing oneself	P					
		C					
d530	Toileting	P					
		C					
d540	Dressing	P					
		C					
d550	Eating	P					
		C					
d560	Drinking	P					
		C					
d850	Remunerative employment	P	9				
		C					

ENVIRONMENTAL FACTORS		Facilitator					Barrier			
		+4	+3	+2	+1	0	1	2	3	4
e115	Products and technology for personal use in daily living									
e120	Products and techn. for pers. indoor and outdoor mobility and transportation									
e310	Immediate family									
e340	Personal care providers and personal assistants					9				
e355	Health professionals									

Figure 14.
Functioning profile of a person with a spinal cord injury in post-acute care (Brief version)

Note. In Body Functions, Body Structures, Activities and Participation: 0 = no problem, 1 = mild problem, 2 = moderate problem, 3 = severe problem, 4 = complete problem; In Environmental Factors: 0 = no barrier/facilitator, 1 = mild barrier, 2 = moderate barrier, 3 = severe barrier, 4 = complete barrier, +1 = mild facilitator, +2 = moderate facilitator, +3 = substantial facilitator, +4 = complete facilitator, 8 = not specified, 9 = not applicable

P = Performance, C = Capacity

5.2.6. Discussion – Implementing ICF Core Sets in Interdisciplinary Settings

The ICF makes it possible to use the ICF Core Sets as a multidimensional tool for the description of functioning by integrating ICF categories from Body Functions, Body Structures, Activities and Participation, and Environmental Factors. This ICF multidimensional framework allows different professionals who are experts in distinct fields of health care provision to systematically collect and structure comprehensive information.

For interdisciplinary rehabilitation planning, the assessment of functioning and the impact of the environment have to be comprehensive and detailed. To meet this need, users are encouraged either to select the Enlarged Brief version or the Comprehensive ICF Core Set. To apply the Enlarged Brief version, the user has to select ICF categories from the Comprehensive ICF Core Set that are not included in the Brief version to perform a more detailed description of functioning. This requires an additional selection process and, more importantly, sufficient knowledge of the user regarding the potential problems in functioning related to a particular health condition. The Comprehensive ICF Core Set already includes the full list of relevant ICF categories and therefore can serve as a reference that can remind the user not to overlook domains of functioning. The Comprehensive ICF Core Set gives the full picture of a person's functioning, but as these sets may have more than 100 ICF categories, the responsibility for describing the individual ICF categories should be distributed among members of an interdisciplinary team.

In this use case, the ICF Core Set was applied to a patient suffering from SCI during the first rehabilitation. SCI is one example of a health condition in which patients are faced with manifold problems related to their level of functioning. To provide optimal care, an interdisciplinary approach should include the patient and his family.[76] The basis for optimal management of SCI is an in-depth and systematic understanding and sound measurement of the problems in functioning.[77] This understanding needs also to be shared by all persons involved in care management.

To identify and address the patient's manifold needs and to be able to compare his level of functioning over time for interdisciplinary rehabilitation planning, the Comprehensive ICF Core Set for SCI in Post-Acute Care was selected. This ICF Core Set includes 162 ICF categories, 104 2nd-, 49 3rd- and 9 4th-level categories. The high total number of ICF categories and, in particular, the high number of 3rd- and 4th-level categories facilitates a very detailed description of functioning. Applying the Comprehensive ICF Core Set ensures that all potential problems and needs will be identified and that the information will be sufficient for rehabilitation planning.

The responsibility of performing the required comprehensive assessment in this use case was distributed among the team members. The team consisted of a rehabilitation psychiatrist, nurses, physical, sport and occupational therapists, a psychologist and social workers, including a vocational counsellor. Table 7 shows who was responsible for each ICF category:

All team members were involved in some feature of the description of functioning. While for some ICF categories more than one professional was involved in the assessment, only one was responsible for the rating of the problem (marked with bold and capital X). The distribution among team members contributed to the creation of a comprehensive picture of the patient's functioning while at the same time using human resources in an optimal way.

This use case illustrates the application of the Comprehensive ICF Core Set in an interdisciplinary team for rehabilitation management. The use of Comprehensive ICF Core Sets facilitates the depiction of the full picture of a person's functioning. However, due to the high number of ICF categories of the Comprehensive Core Sets, their application is useful in interdisciplinary teams only when the responsibilities for the description can be distributed among team members.

Table 7.
Distribution of responsibilities among interdisciplinary team (illustration of all categories from the Brief ICF Core Set and selected ICF categories from the Comprehensive ICF Core Set for SCI in Post-Acute Care)

		Phys	Nurse	PT	OT	Sport	Psych	SW
b130	Energy and drive functions	x					**X**	
b134	Sleep functions		**X**					
b152	Emotional functions						**X**	
b280	Sensation of pain	**X**	x	x				
b440	Respiration functions	**X**						
b525	Defecation functions	**X**	x					
b620	Urination functions	**X**	x					
b730	Muscle power functions			**X**	x			
b735	Muscle tone functions	**X**		x				
b810	Protective functions of the skin		**X**					
s120	Spinal cord and related structures	**X**						
s430	Structure of respiratory system	**X**						
s610	Structure of urinary system	**X**						
d230	Carrying out daily routine		**X**					
d410	Changing basic body position		x	**X**	x			
d420	Transferring oneself		x	**X**	x			
d445	Hand and arm use			x	**X**			
d450	Walking			**X**				
d455	Moving around			**X**				
d465	Moving around using equipment			x	x	X		
d510	Washing oneself		**X**		x			
d530	Toileting		**X**		x			
d540	Dressing		**X**		x			
d550	Eating		**X**					
d560	Drinking		**X**					
d850	Remunerative employment							**X**
d920	Recreation and leisure					**X**		x
e115	Products and technology for personal use in daily living		**X**		x			
e120	Products and technology for personal indoor and outdoor mobility and transportation			x	**X**			
e310	Immediate family	x	x				x	**X**
e340	Personal care providers and personal assistants							**X**
e355	Health professionals	**X**						
e570	Social security services, systems and policies							**X**

Note. All categories from the Generic Set are also integrated. The main responsibilities are highlighted in grey boxes.
Phys = physiatrist, PT = physical therapist, OT = occupational therapist, Sport = sport therapist, SW = social worker

5.3. Use Case 3: Applying the ICF Core Set for Multiple Sclerosis in Long-Term Care

Andrea Glässel and Miriam Lückenkemper

This use case illustrates the application of an ICF Core Set for a patient with chronic multiple sclerosis (MS) being treated in an interdisciplinary setting in an inpatient rehabilitation centre. It also discusses how ICF-based documentation can be used to describe, not just patient problems, but patient resources.

5.3.1. The Case

Mrs. Campalla is a 62-year-old woman. Years ago, early symptoms of MS disease (ICD-10: G35)[8] began, and a year later the diagnosis of MS was confirmed. At the beginning, her disease had appeared to be taking primarily a relapsing course, but recently it is increasingly taking on a chronic-progressive form of the disease. On the Expanded Disability Status Scale (EDSS)[78] she scored 6.0 out of 10.0. Mrs. Campalla is retired and lives with her husband in a house with stairs and an external elevator. She has never been in neurological inpatient rehabilitation, but she has been regularly treated in an outpatient physical therapy setting for some years. On admission to the rehabilitation centre, she exhibited a spastic-ataxic syndrome predominant in the right leg. She was able to walk a maximum distance of 100 meters using a walker and a splint for her right ankle and her gait pattern was stabilized with hyperextension of her right knee. She described her problems mainly as movement restrictions and did not report restrictions in mental and cognitive functions. Mrs. Campalla has an optimistic and positive attitude towards the future and is highly motivated to follow her treatment plan, works well with therapists and performs her rehabilitation exercises intensively.

Mrs. Campalla's overall rehabilitation goal is to live independently at home with the support of her husband and her caregiver. Physical therapists concentrated on improving her walking safety and training her balance and muscle strength in the lower extremities. She had intensive pelvic floor training to improve impaired micturition of her bladder. Occupational therapists assessed her functioning in carrying out her daily routine and, to increase her autonomy, they focused on self-care, dressing and her abilities to care for the household. Mrs. Campalla is able to perform these activities on her own. Although she needs more time to complete an activity, she has developed compensation strategies for her independence. She was able to walk more than 10 meters under supervision but now can do so without a walker by using a splint for her ankle. After three weeks in rehabilitation, Mrs. Campalla was discharged home. To maintain her functioning level, the interdisciplinary team of the rehabilitation centre recommended the continuation of outpatient physical therapy and exercises.

5.3.2. The Application Area and Setting

Mrs. Campalla has been treated in an inpatient rehabilitation centre that specializes in MS. The centre offers different approaches to rehabilitation management for neurological conditions, from comprehensive inpatient rehabilitation management in the early post-acute context to outpatient rehabilitative interventions in the long-term. Inpatient rehabilitation management is provided by an interdisciplinary team that addresses the MS needs of the patient from a holistic perspective. The interdisciplinary team consists of physical therapists, occupational therapists, physicians, nurses, neuropsychologists and sport therapists, who, together with Mrs. Campalla, developed a treatment plan to achieve defined rehabilitation goals.

5.3.3. The Purpose of Applying an ICF Core Set

To describe the patient's level of functioning fully from the perspectives of the interdisciplinary team, the ICF Core Set was applied for treatment planning and evaluation. The team used the ICF categories of the ICF Core Set for assessment and for evaluation and preparing the discharge report, which will be sent to Mrs. Campalla's outpatient physical therapist.

5.3.4 Selection of the Appropriate ICF Core Set

The selection of the appropriate ICF Core Set was performed in two steps: selection of the health condition-related or condition group-related ICF Core Set and selection of the appropriate types of ICF Core Sets (Figure 15).

Choice of ICF Core Set Related to Specific Health Condition or Condition Group

To describe this patient's functioning and level of disability, the ICF Core Set for MS in Long-Term Care[30] was selected. ICF Core Sets serve to structure the information obtained in terms of the biopsychosocial model of the ICF and therefore

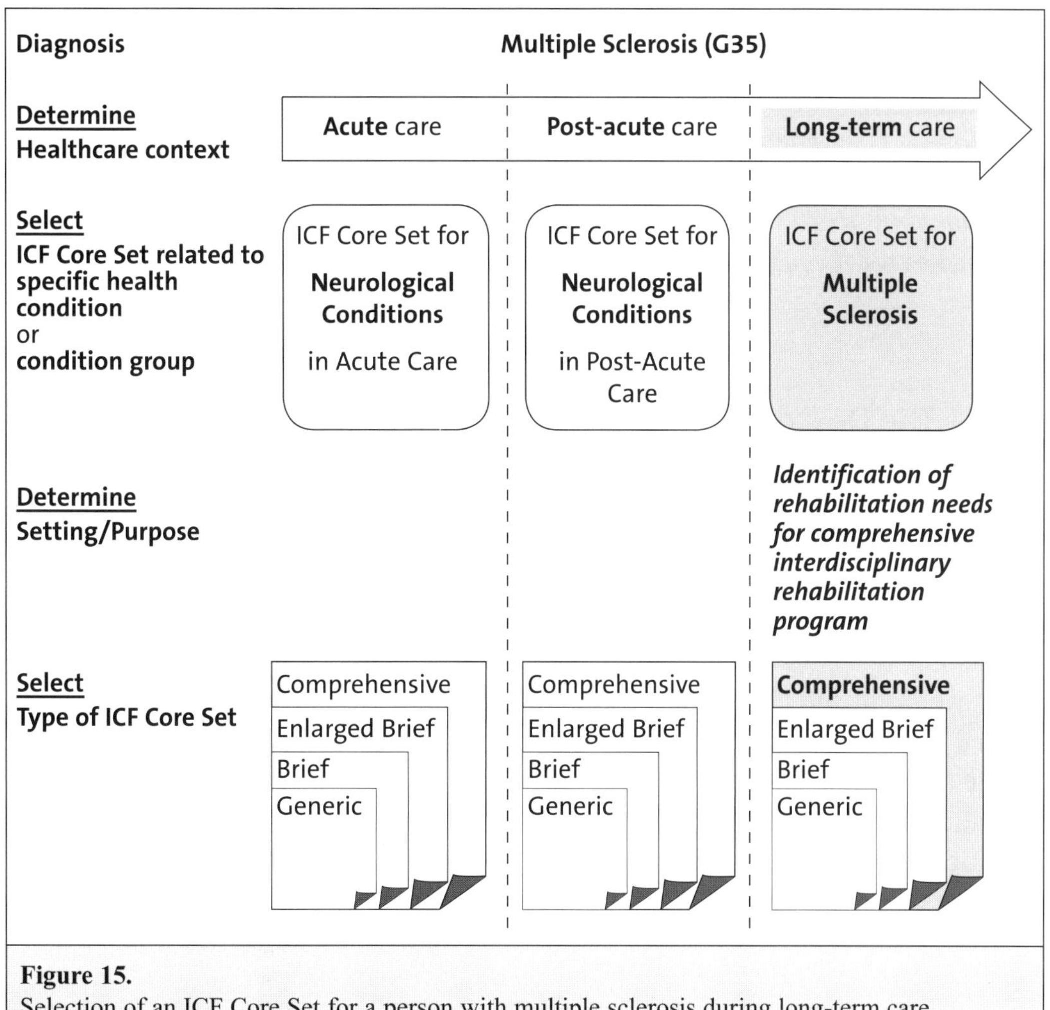

Figure 15.
Selection of an ICF Core Set for a person with multiple sclerosis during long-term care

to guide the treatment and rehabilitation process.[30] The Comprehensive ICF Core Set for MS includes 138 2nd- and 3rd-level ICFcategories (40 Body Functions, 7 Body Structures, 53 Activities and Participation categories and 38 Environmental Factors). The Brief ICF Core Set for MS includes 19 2nd-level ICF categories (8 Body Functions, 2 Body Structures, 5 Activities and Participation categories, 4 Environmental Factors).

Choice of Type of ICF Core Set

To describe Mrs. Campalla's level of functioning and disability, the Enlarged Brief version was used, resulting in a combination of 49 ICF categories from the different types of the ICF Core Set for MS. As recommended, the category from the Generic Set not available in the Brief ICF Core Set for MS, namely *d455 Moving around,* was added to the Brief ICF Core Set. To increase the comprehensiveness of the Brief ICF Core Set, six additional categories were selected from the Comprehensive ICF Core Set for MS (*b140 Attention function, b144 Memory functions, b735 Muscle tone functions, d170 Writing, d920 Recreation and Leisure, e1101 Drugs),* resulting in a total of 49 ICF categories for the documentation form.

5.3.5. The Description of Functioning with the Documentation Form

To fill in the documentation form, information was gathered from Mrs. Campalla's case history, medical reports from the health professionals, technical investigations and a patient interview. Clinical examinations were also performed on several areas of functioning. The available information was rated afterwards using the ICF qualifiers in light of the clinical experience of the physical therapist. The results were entered in the documentation form below (Figure 16), from which the functioning profile (Figure 17) was created. Both figures present the brief version of the documentation form and the functioning profile (consisting of all ICF categories from the Brief ICF Core Set for MS combined with the Generic Set). The full version is available on the CD included in the Manual.

BODY FUNCTIONS = physiological functions of body systems (including psychological functions) ***How much impairment does the person have in...***		No impairment	Mild impairment	Moderate impairment	Severe impairment	Complete impairment	Not specified	Not applicable
b130	**Energy and drive functions**	0	**1**	2	3	4	8	9
	General mental functions of physiological and psychological mechanisms that cause the individual to move towards satisfying specific needs and general goals in a persistent manner. *Inclusions: functions of energy level, motivation, appetite, craving (including craving for substances that can be abused), and impulse control* *Exclusions: consciousness functions (b110); temperament and personality functions (b126); sleep functions (b134); psychomotor functions (b147); emotional functions (b152)*							
	Sources of information: ☒ Case history ☐ Patient-reported questionnaire ☐ Clinical examination ☐ Technical investigation							
	Description of the problem: *She was very motivated and engaged to participate in treatment and therapy, is performing exercises by herself.*							

Figure 16. Continued on next page

b152	Emotional functions	0	**1**	2	3	4	8	9
	Specific mental functions related to the feeling and affective components of the processes of the mind. *Inclusions: functions of appropriateness of emotion, regulation and range of emotion; affect; sadness, happiness, love, fear, anger, hate, tension, anxiety, joy, sorrow; lability of emotion; flattening of affect* *Exclusions: temperament and personality functions (b126); energy and drive functions (b130)*							
	Sources of information: ☒ Case history ☐ Patient-reported questionnaire ☐ Clinical examination ☐ Technical investigation							
	Description of the problem: *Sometimes she has mood fluctuations.*							
b164	Higher-level cognitive functions	**0**	1	2	3	4	8	9
	Specific mental functions especially dependent on the frontal lobes of the brain, including complex goal-directed behaviours such as decision-making, abstract thinking, planning and carrying out plans, mental flexibility, and deciding which behaviours are appropriate under what circumstances; often called executive functions. *Inclusions: functions of abstraction and organization of ideas; time management, insight and judgement; concept formation, categorization and cognitive flexibility* *Exclusions: memory functions (b144); thought functions (b160); mental functions of language (b167); calculation functions (b172)*							
	Sources of information: ☒ Case history ☐ Patient-reported questionnaire ☐ Clinical examination ☐ Technical investigation							
	Description of the problem: –							
b210	Seeing functions	0	**1**	2	3	4	8	9
	Sensory functions relating to sensing the presence of light and sensing the form, size, shape and colour of the visual stimuli. *Inclusions: visual acuity functions; visual field functions; quality of vision; functions of sensing light and colour, visual acuity of distant and near vision, monocular and binocular vision; visual picture quality; impairments such as myopia, hypermetropia, astigmatism, hemianopia, colour-blindness, tunnel vision, central and peripheral scotoma, diplopia, night blindness and impaired adaptability to light* *Exclusion: perceptual functions (b156)*							
	Sources of information: ☒ Case history ☐ Patient-reported questionnaire ☒ Clinical examination ☒ Technical investigation							
	Description of the problem: *Slight fuzziness in her vision (no diplopic images). Glasses are required for reading.*							
b280	Sensation of pain	0	1	**2**	3	4	8	9
	Sensation of unpleasant feeling indicating potential or actual damage to some body structure. *Inclusions: sensations of generalized or localized pain in one or more body part, pain in a dermatome, stabbing pain, burning pain, dull pain, aching pain; impairments such as myalgia, analgesia and hyperalgesia*							
	Sources of information: ☐ Case history ☐ Patient-reported questionnaire ☒ Clinical examination ☐ Technical investigation							
	Description of the problem: *Visual Analog Scale (VAS) Score 4 emissive in low back pain and the right leg.*							

Figure 16. Continued on next page

b620	Urination functions	0	1	**2**	3	4	8	9
	Functions of discharge of urine from the urinary bladder. *Inclusions: functions of urination, frequency of urination, urinary continence; impairments such as in stress, urge, reflex, overflow, continuous incontinence, dribbling, automatic bladder, polyuria, urinary retention and urinary urgency* *Exclusions: urinary excretory functions (b610); sensations associated with urinary functions (b630)*							
	Sources of information: ☒ Case history ☐ Patient-reported questionnaire ☒ Clinical examination ☐ Technical investigation							
	Description of the problem: *She has problems in urination due to spastic bladder; patient is drinking too little liquid per day. Recurrent bladder infections connected with pain (not at present).*							
b730	Muscle power functions	0	1	**2**	3	4	8	9
	Functions related to the force generated by the contraction of a muscle or muscle groups. *Inclusions: functions associated with the power of specific muscles and muscle groups, muscles of one limb, one side of the body, the lower half of the body, all limbs, the trunk and the body as a whole; impairments such as weakness of small muscles in feet and hands, muscle paresis, muscle paralysis, monoplegia, hemiplegia, paraplegia, quadriplegia and akinetic mutism* *Exclusions: functions of structures adjoining the eye (b215); muscle tone functions (b735); muscle endurance functions (b740)*							
	Sources of information: ☒ Case history ☐ Patient-reported questionnaire ☒ Clinical examination ☐ Technical investigation							
	Description of the problem: *Manual muscle testing (MMM) was performed for muscles relevant for gait patterns* *Decreased force in her right femoral and hip muscles, especially by making squats for example sitting down on a chair.*							

	left	right
M. Iliopsoas	5	4
M. glutaeus maximus	4	4
M. glutaei med./min.	4	3
M. ischiocrurale	5	4
M. quadriceps	4	3
M. tibialis anterior	4	2

b770	Gait pattern functions	0	1	2	**3**	4	8	9
	Functions of movement patterns associated with walking, running or other whole body movements. *Inclusions: walking patterns and running patterns; impairments such as spastic gait, hemiplegic gait, paraplegic gait, asymmetric gait, limping and stiff gait pattern* *Exclusions: muscle power functions (b730); muscle tone functions (b735); control of voluntary movement functions (b760); involuntary movement functions (b765)*							
	Sources of information: ☒ Case history ☐ Patient-reported questionnaire ☒ Clinical examination ☐ Technical investigation							
	Description of the problem: *Hyperextending right knee during walking; club foot (pes equinus).*							

Figure 16. Continued on next page

BODY STRUCTURES = anatomical parts of the body such as organs, limbs and their components ***How much impairment does the person have in the...***			**No impairment**		**Mild impairment**		**Moderate impairment**		**Severe impairment**		**Complete impairment**		**Not specified**	**Not applicable**
s110	**Structure of brain**	**Extent**	0		1		2		3		4		8	9
		Nature*	0		1	2	3	4	5	6	7		8	9
		Location**	0		1	2	3	4	5	6	7		8	9

Sources of information:
☐ Case history ☐ Patient-reported questionnaire ☐ Clinical examination ☐ Technical investigation

Description of the problem:
X-ray not available

s120	**Spinal cord and related structures**	**Extent**	0		1		2		3		4		8	9
		Nature*	0		1	2	3	4	5	6	7		8	9
		Location**	0		1	2	3	4	5	6	7		8	9

Sources of information:
☒ Case history ☐ Patient-reported questionnaire ☐ Clinical examination ☐ Technical investigation

Description of the problem:
X-ray / MRI not available.

ACTIVITIES AND PARTICIPATION = execution of a task or action by an individual and involvement in a life situation ***How much difficulty does the person have in the...*** ***P = performance of...*** ***C = capacity in...***			**No difficulty**	**Mild difficulty**	**Moderate difficulty**	**Severe difficulty**	**Complete difficulty**	**Not specified**	**Not applicable**
d175	**Solving problems**	**P**	0	1	2	3	4	8	9
		C	0	1	2	3	4	8	9

Finding solutions to questions or situations by identifying and analysing issues, developing options and solutions, evaluating potential effects of solutions and executing a chosen solution, such as in resolving a dispute between two people.
Inclusions: solving simple and complex problems
Exclusions: thinking (d163); making decisions (d177)

Sources of information:
☒ Case history ☐ Patient-reported questionnaire ☐ Clinical examination ☐ Technical investigation

Description of the problem:
P: *No problems in adequately solving problems observed.*
C: *No standard test setting used.*

Figure 16. Continued on next page

d230	Carrying out daily routine							
	P	0	1	**2**	3	4	8	9
	C	0	1	2	3	4	**8**	9

Carrying out simple or complex and coordinated actions in order to plan, manage and complete the requirements of day-to-day procedures or duties, such as budgeting time and making plans for separate activities throughout the day.
Inclusions: managing and completing the daily routine; managing one's own activity level
Exclusion: undertaking multiple tasks (d220)

Sources of information:

☒ Case history ☐ Patient-reported questionnaire ☒ Clinical examination ☐ Technical investigation

Description of the problem:

P: *Managing daily routine at her own pace; patient takes more time / treatment indicated (need of breaks).*
C: *No standardized test available.*

d450	Walking							
	P	0	1	**2**	3	4	8	9
	C	0	1	2	**3**	4	8	9

Moving along a surface on foot, step by step, so that one foot is always on the ground, such as when strolling, sauntering, walking forwards, backwards or sideways.
Inclusions: walking short or long distances; walking on different surfaces; walking around obstacles
Exclusions: transferring oneself (d420); moving around (d455)

Sources of information:

☒ Case history ☐ Patient-reported questionnaire ☒ Clinical examination ☐ Technical investigation

Description of the problem:

P: *walking short distances with walker and splints possible in her own pace; takes more time, increased attention; 100 meters EDSS: 6.0*
C: *She is able to walk without assistive devices (splint and walker) 5–10 step.*

d455∞	Moving around							
	P	0	1	2	**3**	4	8	9
	C	0	1	2	3	**4**	8	9

Moving the whole body from one place to another by means other than walking, such as climbing over a rock or running down a street, skipping, scampering, jumping, somersaulting or running around obstacles.
Inclusions: crawling, climbing, running, jogging, jumping, and swimming
Exclusions: transferring oneself (d420); walking (d450)

Sources of information:

☒ Case history ☐ Patient-reported questionnaire ☒ Clinical examination ☐ Technical investigation

Description of the problem:

P: *Moving around at her own pace and with a walker and splint; takes more time and increased attention; outside with uneven floor is difficult for her; 100 meters with a walker and splint.*
C: *She is not able to walk outside without walker and splint.*

Figure 16. Continued on next page

d760	**Family relationships**	P	0	1	2	3	4	8	9
		C	0	1	2	3	4	8	9
	Creating and maintaining kinship relationships, such as with members of the nuclear family, extended family, foster and adopted family and step-relationships, more distant relationships such as second cousins or legal guardians. *Inclusions: parent-child and child-parent relationships, sibling and extended family relationships*								
	Sources of information: ☒ Case history ☐ Patient-reported questionnaire ☒ Clinical examination ☐ Technical investigation								
	Description of the problem: *P:* – *C:* –								
d850	**Remunerative employment**	P	0	1	2	3	4	8	9
		C	0	1	2	3	4	8	9
	Engaging in all aspects of work, as an occupation, trade, profession or other form of employment, for payment, as an employee, full or part time, or self-employed, such as seeking employment and getting a job, doing the required tasks of the job, attending work on time as required, supervising other workers or being supervised, and performing required tasks alone or in groups. *Inclusions: self-employment, part-time and full-time employment*								
	Sources of information: ☐ Case history ☐ Patient-reported questionnaire ☐ Clinical examination ☐ Technical investigation								
	Description of the problem: ***P + C:*** *Patient is retired.*								

ENVIRONMENTAL FACTORS = make up the physical, social and attitudinal environment in which people live and conduct their lives ***How much of a facilitator or barrier does the person experience with respect to...***		Complete facilitator	Substantial facilitator	Moderate facilitator	Mild facilitator	No barrier/facilitator	Mild barrier	Moderate barrier	Substantial barrier	Complete barrier	Not specified	Not applicable
e310	**Immediate family**	+4	+3	+2	+1	0	1	2	3	4	8	9
	Individuals related by birth, marriage or other relationship recognized by the culture as immediate family, such as spouses, partners, parents, siblings, children, foster parents, adoptive parents and grandparents. *Exclusions: extended family (e315); personal care providers and personal assistants (e340)*											
	Sources of information: ☒ Case history ☐ Patient-reported questionnaire ☐ Clinical examination ☐ Technical investigation											
	Description of the facilitator/barrier: *Her husband is most important; he supports her any time she needs him.*											

Figure 16. Continued on next page

e355	Health professionals	**+4**	+3	+2	+1	0	1	2	3	4	8	9

All service providers working within the context of the health system, such as doctors, nurses, physiotherapists, occupational therapists, speech therapists, audiologists, orthotist-prosthetists, medical social workers.
Exclusion: other professionals (e360)

Sources of information:

☒ Case history ☐ Patient-reported questionnaire ☐ Clinical examination ☐ Technical investigation

Description of the facilitator/barrier:

Receives support from the medical doctor and gets outpatient treatment from a physical therapist.

e410	Individual attitudes of immediate family members	+4	**+3**	+2	+1	0	1	2	3	4	8	9

General or specific opinions and beliefs of immediate family members about the person or about other matters (e.g. social, political and economic issues) that influence individual behaviour and actions.

Sources of information:

☒ Case history ☐ Patient-reported questionnaire ☐ Clinical examination ☐ Technical investigation

Description of the facilitator/barrier:

Positive attitudes of the family.

e580	Health services, systems and policies	+4	**+3**	+2	+1	0	1	2	3	4	8	9

Services, systems and policies for preventing and treating health problems, providing medical rehabilitation and promoting a healthy lifestyle.
Exclusion: general social support services, systems and policies (e575)

Sources of information:

☒ Case history ☐ Patient-reported questionnaire ☐ Clinical examination ☐ Technical investigation

Description of the facilitator/barrier:

Rehabilitation stay was completely paid by the health insurance; outpatient treatment is fully covered by the health insurance.

PERSONAL FACTORS

The patient had an optimistic and positive attitude about the future. She was very highly motivated to follow her training plan and work diligently with her therapists.

She has developed strategies to cope with her situation.

Figure 16.
ICF Core Set based documentation form based on the ICF Core Set for Multiple Sclerosis (Brief version)

Note. ICF categories marked in dark grey belong to the Generic Set and are included in any documentation form

∞ Category from the Generic Set not included in the ICF Core Set for Multiple Sclerosis

* Rating of the nature of the impairment in Body Structures: 0 = no change in structure, 1 = total absence, 2 = partial absence, 3 = additional part, 4 = aberrant dimension, 5 = discontinuity, 6 = deviating position, 7 = qualitative changes in structure, 8 = not specified, 9 = not applicable

** Rating of the location of the impairment in Body Structures: 0 = more than one region, 1 = right, 2 = left, 3 = both sides, 4 = front, 5 = back, 6 = proximal, 7 = distal, 8 = not specified, 9 = not applicable

BODY FUNCTIONS		Impairment				
		0	1	2	3	4
b130	Energy and drive functions					
b152	Emotional functions					
b164	Higher-level cognitive functions					
b210	Seeing functions					
b280	Sensation of pain					
b620	Urination functions					
b730	Muscle power functions					
b770	Gait pattern functions					

BODY STRUCTURES		Impairment				
		0	1	2	3	4
s110	Structure of brain	8				
s120	Spinal cord and related structures	8				

ACTIVITIES AND PARTICIPATION			Difficulty				
			0	1	2	3	4
d175	Solving problems	P					
		C	8				
d230	Carrying out daily routine	P					
		C	8				
d450	Walking	P					
		C					
d455∞	Moving around	P					
		C					
d760	Family relationships	P					
		C					
d850	Remunerative employment	P	9				
		C	9				

ENVIRONMENTAL FACTORS		Facilitator					Barrier			
		+4	+3	+2	+1	0	1	2	3	4
e310	Immediate family									
e355	Health professionals									
e410	Individual attitudes of immediate family members									
e580	Health services, systems and policies									

Figure 17.
Functioning profile of a person with multiple sclerosis in long-term care

Note. In Body Functions, Body Structures, Activities and Participation: 0 = no problem, 1 = mild problem, 2 = moderate problem, 3 = severe problem, 4 = complete problem; In Environmental Factors: 0 = no barrier/facilitator, 1 = mild barrier, 2 = moderate barrier, 3 = severe barrier, 4 = complete barrier, +1 = mild facilitator, +2 = moderate facilitator, +3 = substantial facilitator, +4 = complete facilitator, 8 = not specified, 9 = not applicable

P = Performance, C = Capacity

∞ ICF category from the Generic Set not included in the ICF Core Set for Multiple Sclerosis

5.3.6 Discussion – Describing Patient Resources with the ICF Core Set-Based Documentation Form

Patient resources play an important role in the rehabilitation process and contribute to the rehabilitation outcome. Patient resources cover a broad spectrum of factors: from positive attitudes and optimism in life situations, self-confidence and motivation to a body that is fit enough to overcome illness and relationships that are supportive and encouraging. Available resources of these sorts enable a person to handle difficult life situations or cope with a chronic disease like MS.[79–80] The ICF has the advantage of making it possible to describe personal resources in various ways. Three of these approaches are described below.

Firstly, to describe the patient's resources in the context of functioning, the qualifier "0" is crucial. In contrast to using the qualifier scale from "1 to 4" when describing disability, full functioning is expressed by using the qualifier 0 "No problem". In this manner the absence of a problem can be denoted as a patient resource. This is exemplified in the documentation form for this use case by the notation for the ICF category *b130 Energy and drive functions* with the additional comment "she was very motivated and engaged to participate in treatment and therapy".

Secondly, the patient's external resources can be described as facilitators in the Environmental Factors of the ICF on the qualifier scale from "+1 to +4" (see Chapter 2). The strength of the use of ICF Core Sets is that they make resources transparent by identifying facilitators, while many assessment tools in MS such as the EDSS[78] focus entirely on the description of problems. Since the ICF also allows for the description of environmental barriers, these can be clearly analyzed and, with appropriate interventions, can potentially be transformed into resources. In the present case, Mrs Campalla had the steps in her house substituted by an elevator (e150).

Thirdly, the patient's internal resources are included in Personal Factors, which, though not classified, can be described and added at the end of the documentation form to complete a comprehensive description of the individual. Personal Factors can be a fundamental resource that may influence the patient's functioning in a positive manner. Examples such as "interest in or motivation for training" or "coping strategies to perform activities of daily living" are crucial for a positive outcome in rehabilitation and should be taken into account by health professionals. Compensation strategies such as "taking breaks when required" or "planning more time for dressing without assistance" are resources that enable a person to do an activity independently. Finally, the personal factor "positive attitude to increased time consumption" is also an important patient resource.

In summary, the ICF facilitates the description of personal resources and consequently contributes to their consideration for treatment planning. Integrating patient resources facilitates patient-oriented management and so positively affects treatment strategies and helps to secure rehabilitation outcomes. The documentation form offers the possibility of identifying patient resources across all domains of functioning and contextual factors. This provides a broad picture of the patient's problems and needs, as well as, in particular, the patient's resources.

5.4. Use Case 4: Applying the ICF Core Set for Vocational Rehabilitation in Long-Term Care

Monika Finger and Miriam Lückenkemper

This use case illustrates the application of an ICF Core Set to a person who has been admitted to a vocational rehabilitation programme. It also discusses challenges in rating capacity and performance for levels of functioning in the Activities and Participation component.

5.4.1. The Case

Mrs. Wilson is a 39-year-old landscape gardener whose work is rather heavy and physically challenging and involves difficult forced positions of the trunk and spine as well as overhead work. Twelve months ago Mrs. Wilson had a work accident falling from a ladder while cutting a tree. She suffered a disc herniation between 6th and 7th cervical vertebrae (ICD 10: S13.0) and fractures of the 5th and 6th thoracic vertebrae (ICD 10: S22.1) both without compression of the spinal cord. She was off from work for 12 months after the accident and she is currently suffering from adjustment disorder and shows a continuing depressive reaction (ICD 10:F43.2). Mrs. Wilson is divorced and lives with a new partner and her 12-year-old son in a four-room apartment with a terrace and a small garden.

After an intensive multimodal rehabilitation programme, including work conditioning interventions, exercise training and psychological coaching, physicians recommended that she change her profession. The treating physicians assessed Mrs. Wilson as having a full work capacity for light work. According to the DOT system (Dictionary of Occupational Titles) light work is defined as follows: "Requires the ability to stand up to six hours in an eight-hour work day, lift up to 10 pounds frequently and up to 20 pounds occasionally".[81]

5.4.2. The Application Setting

The setting for this use case is one in which vocational rehabilitation (VR) is offered. VR can be defined as "a multi-professional evidence-based approach that is provided in different settings, services and activities to working age individuals with health-related impairments, limitations or restrictions with work functioning, and whose primary aim is to optimize work participation".[82]

Currently, Mrs. Wilson is taking part in a vocational rehabilitation programme at a rehabilitation centre in order to evaluate her level of functioning for light work. She attends an outpatient program five days a week during which a team of vocational consultants and coaches, together with social workers and psychologists, comprehensively evaluate her physical and mental status. This four week standard evaluation consists of testing her abilities and assessing her resources and aims to describe these abilities as completely as possible in order to decide on an appropriate working position. During this program, vocational professionals will also clarify her financial situation and identify potential funding sources for a job change or a new professional education. Together with Mrs. Wilson, the vocational team is looking for occupational retraining, on-the-job training or an apprenticeship. Medical treatment or physical therapy and training are only provided during the programme when they are necessary.

5.4.3. The Purpose of Applying an ICF Core Set

An ICF Core Set can make it possible for the health professionals to describe Mrs. Wilson's functioning situation in a structured and standardized way. This enables health care service providers from different health professions to set up a common functioning profile so that members of the interdisciplinary team can coordinate interventions and rehabilitation management. In addition, Mrs. Wilson will be better informed about vocational opportunities and she can find the best possible work solution together with her vocational counsellors.

5.4.4. Selection of the Appropriate ICF Core Set

The selection of the appropriate ICF Core Set was performed in two steps: selection of the health condition-related or condition group-related ICF Core Set and selection of the appropriate type of ICF Core Set (Figure 18).

Choice of ICF Core Set Related to Specific Health Condition or Condition Group

Unlike other ICF Core Sets, the ICF Core Set for VR is independent of the health condition and applies to any setting where vocational rehabilitation is provided.[60] In most cases, the ICF Core Set for VR will be applied in the post-acute or long-term context[58] since VR or occupational reintegration are provided when the client's acute

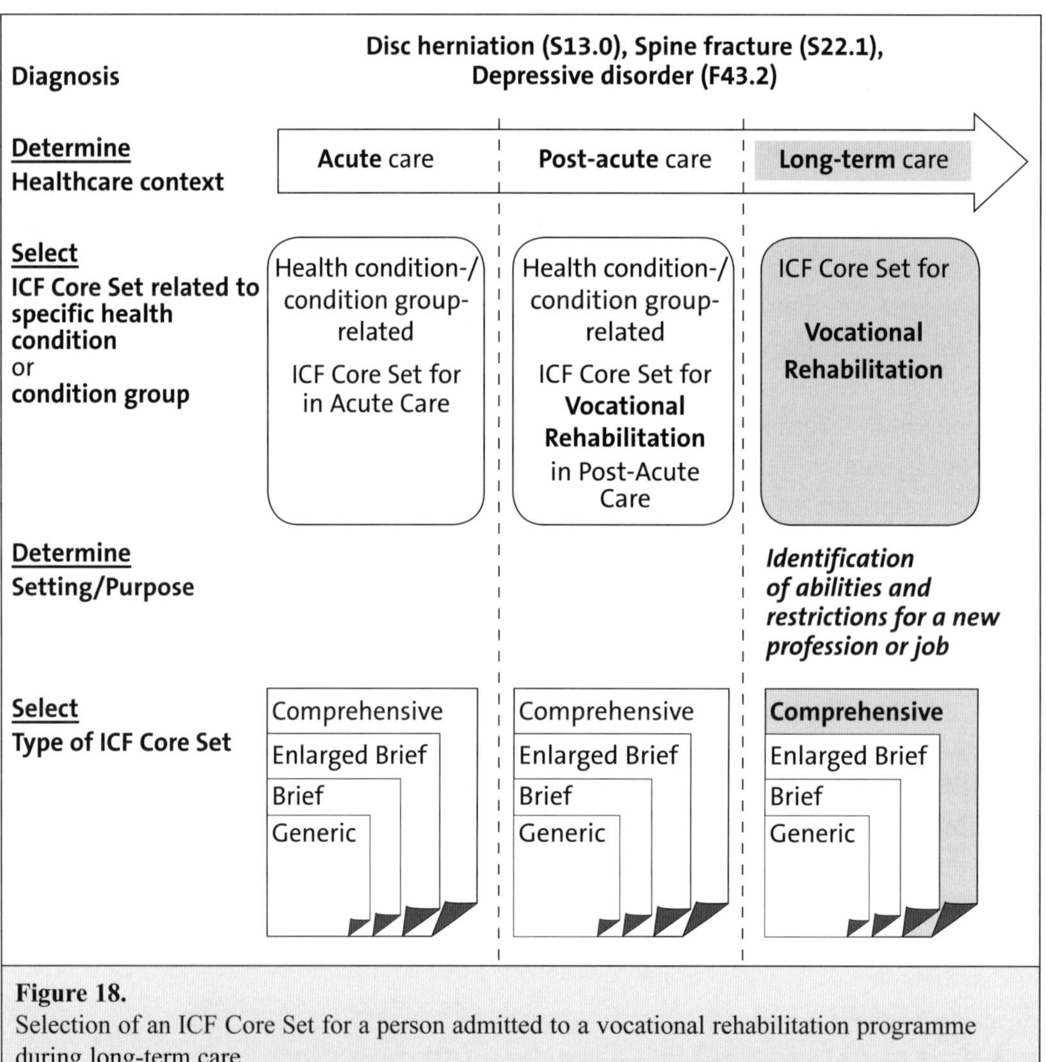

Figure 18.
Selection of an ICF Core Set for a person admitted to a vocational rehabilitation programme during long-term care

physical or mental state has stabilized. In the acute phase, and sometimes also in the post-acute phase, the ICF Core Set for VR may be selected in addition to a relevant health condition-related or condition group related Core Set.

Choice of Type of ICF Core Set

VR is a very complex process and often involves multiple health care professionals and settings and also takes into account the workplace environment. Along the continuum of VR, an ICF Core Set can be used for different purposes. In particular, it can be used as a checklist to assess and document problems in functioning and to identify environmental facilitators and barriers in a standardized way. Using a common standard such as the ICF Core Set for VR can also enhance communication between the vocational rehabilitation specialists and other professionals or when the client is changing the health care or rehabilitation setting.

The *Brief Core Set for VR* is useful for assessing the overall situation of a client group or for describing a study population. However, for the interdisciplinary clinical context, the Brief Core Set will not be sufficient in some situations. The *Comprehensive ICF Core Set for VR* includes 90 categories (89 2nd-level and one 3rd-level category, *e1101 Drugs*). Forty categories are from the Activities and Participation component, 33 from Environmental Factors and 17 categories from Body Functions. No category from Body Structures is included.

In this case, the *Comprehensive ICF Core Set for VR*[58] was selected to create a complete profile of Mrs. Wilson's functioning in relation to her work. As recommended, the Generic Set should be included in the description of a person's functioning, although in this case the Comprehensive ICF Core Set for VR already included the Generic Set categories. This comprehensive profile makes it possible for the health professionals, as well as Mrs. Wilson herself, to reflect on resources and problems when considering new professional perspectives. In addition, the profile may be used to formulate rehabilitation goals when a lack of knowledge and/or skills for a particular job is detected.

5.4.5. The Description of Functioning with the Documentation Form

To apply the ICF Core Sets in this use case, the documentation form contained the 90 categories from the Comprehensive ICF Core Set for VR and was completed based on information taken from Mrs. Wilson's case history, from a patient-reported questionnaire and from clinical examinations. The case history and medical reports reflect the perspective of health professionals and so captured a comprehensive picture of Mrs. Wilson's functioning. The information was entered in the documentation form and rated with the ICF qualifiers by a physical therapist with extensive clinical experience. When rating the areas of functioning in the component Activity and Participation, the distinction between capacity and performance was carefully taken into account. In Mrs. Wilson's situation, a thorough understanding of optimal functioning in real-life situations is particularly required. This is the basis for identifying a suitable profession or job for which Mrs. Wilson can be educated or trained for future employment.

The assessment results of the 90 categories were entered in the documentation form, which provides an overview of the client's weaknesses and strengths and so offers a well-informed basis to steer the process of work reintegration. The documentation form also makes it possible for the interdisciplinary team to start with the required treatment and share intervention strategies. The results are presented in the documentation form below (Figure 19), from which the functioning profile (Figure 20) was created. Both figures present the Brief version of the documentation form and the functioning profile (consisting of all ICF categories from the Brief ICF Core Set for Vocational Rehabilitation and the Generic Set). The full version is available on the CD included with this Manual.

BODY FUNCTIONS = physiological functions of body systems (including psychological functions) ***How much of a problem does the person have in...***		No problem	Mild problem	Moderate problem	Severe problem	Complete problem	Not specified	Not applicable
b130	**Energy and drive functions**	0	1	2	**3** (marked)	4	8	9
	General mental functions of physiological and psychological mechanisms that cause the individual to move towards satisfying specific needs and general goals in a persistent manner. *Inclusions: functions of energy level, motivation, appetite, craving (including craving for substances that can be abused), and impulse control* *Exclusions: consciousness functions (b110); temperament and personality functions (b126); sleep functions (b134); psychomotor functions (b147); emotional functions (b152)*							
	Sources of information: ☒ Case history ☒ Patient-reported questionnaire ☐ Clinical examination ☐ Technical investigation							
	Description of the problem: *Patient reports being limited in her daily activities due to lack of energy.*							
b152	**Emotional functions**	0	1	**2** (marked)	3	4	8	9
	Specific mental functions related to the feeling and affective components of the processes of the mind. *Inclusions: functions of appropriateness of emotion, regulation and range of emotion; affect; sadness, happiness, love, fear, anger, hate, tension, anxiety, joy, sorrow; lability of emotion; flattening of affect* *Exclusions: temperament and personality functions (b126); energy and drive functions (b130)*							
	Sources of information: ☒ Case history ☐ Patient-reported questionnaire ☐ Clinical examination ☐ Technical investigation							
	Description of the problem: *Patient reports anxiety and fear of harming herself. She feels touchy and reacts very fast with anger or tears.*							

Figure 19. Continued on next page

b164	Higher-level cognitive functions	0	**1**	2	3	4	8	9
	Specific mental functions especially dependent on the frontal lobes of the brain, including complex goal-directed behaviours such as decision-making, abstract thinking, planning and carrying out plans, mental flexibility and deciding which behaviours are appropriate under what circumstances; often called executive functions. *Inclusions: functions of abstraction and organization of ideas; time management, insight and judgement; concept formation, categorization and cognitive flexibility* *Exclusions: memory functions (b144); thought functions (b160); mental functions of language (b167); calculation functions (b172)*							
	Sources of information: ☒ Case history ☐ Patient-reported questionnaire ☐ Clinical examination ☐ Technical investigation							
	Description of the problem: *Feels blocked in making decisions and has problems planning and carrying out the things needed to organize her future.*							
b280	Sensation of pain	0	1	2	**3**	4	8	9
	Sensation of unpleasant feeling indicating potential or actual damage to some body structure. *Inclusions: sensations of generalized or localized pain in one or more body part, pain in a dermatome, stabbing pain, burning pain, dull pain, aching pain; impairments such as myalgia, analgesia and hyperalgesia*							
	Sources of information: ☒ Case history ☐ Patient-reported questionnaire ☒ Clinical examination ☐ Technical investigation							
	Description of the problem: *Patient feels a constant pain at rest that elevates to a pain of in the middle of the thoracic spine, when using her arms. When sitting longer than 30min, a pain radiating from her right buttock to her knee arises that forces her to stand up and rest in lying position until pain decreases. Visual Analogue Scale VAS: 3–4/10: at rest, 8–9/10 during movement*							
b455	Exercise tolerance functions	0	1	**2**	3	4	8	9
	Functions related to respiratory and cardiovascular capacity as required for enduring physical exertion. *Inclusions: functions of physical endurance, aerobic capacity, stamina and fatigability* *Exclusions: functions of the cardiovascular system (b410-b429); haematological system functions (b430); respiration functions (b440); respiratory muscle functions (b445); additional respiratory functions (b450)*							
	Sources of information: ☒ Case history ☐ Patient-reported questionnaire ☐ Clinical examination ☐ Technical investigation							
	Description of the problem: *Pace and amount of exercising is diminished due to an increase in fatigue.*							

Figure 19. Continued on next page

ACTIVITIES AND PARTICIPATION = execution of a task or action by an individual and involvement in a life situation *How much of a difficulty does the person have in the...* *P = performance of...* *C = capacity in...*			No difficulty	Mild difficulty	Moderate difficulty	Severe difficulty	Complete difficulty	Not specified	Not applicable
d420	**Acquiring skills**	P	0	1	2	3	4	**8**	9
		C	0	**1**	2	3	4	8	9
	Developing basic and complex competencies in integrated sets of actions or tasks so as to initiate and follow through with the acquisition of a skill, such as manipulating tools or playing games like chess. *Inclusion: acquiring basic and complex skills*								
	Sources of information: ☐ Case history ☐ Patient-reported questionnaire ☒ Clinical examination ☐ Technical investigation								
	Description of the problem: ***P:*** *No information available* ***C:*** *In a basic ability test procedure the ability in learning PC skills is below the norm.*								
d230	**Carrying out daily routine**	P	0	1	**2**	3	4	8	9
		C	0	1	**2**	3	4	8	9
	Carrying out simple or complex and coordinated actions in order to plan, manage and complete the requirements of day-to-day procedures or duties, such as budgeting time and making plans for separate activities throughout the day. *Inclusions: managing and completing the daily routine; managing one's own activity level* *Exclusion: undertaking multiple tasks (d220)*								
	Sources of information: ☒ Case history ☒ Patient-reported questionnaire ☒ Clinical examination ☐ Technical investigation								
	Description of the problem: ***P:*** *Patient reports major problems in fulfilling the needs of her daily life according to the requirements of the household, the VR program and her family because of fatigue and pain.* ***C:*** *In the VR situation it is pointed out that the patient needs more breaks than scheduled and is at her limits in fulfilling the requirements of program.*								
d240	**Handling stress and other psychological demands**	P	0	1	**2**	3	4	8	9
		C	0	**1**	2	3	4	8	9
	Carrying out simple or complex and coordinated actions to manage and control the psychological demands required to carry out tasks demanding significant responsibilities and involving stress, distraction or crises, such as driving a vehicle during heavy traffic or taking care of many children. *Inclusions: handling responsibilities; handling stress and crisis*								
	Sources of information: ☒ Case history ☒ Patient-reported questionnaire ☐ Clinical examination ☐ Technical investigation								
	Description of the problem: ***P:*** *Patient reports that she feels stressed all the time and has major problems to react appropriately in stressful situations.* ***C:*** *No information available*								

Figure 19. Continued on next page

d450	Walking	P	0	1	**2**	3	4	8	9
		C	0	**1**	2	3	4	8	9

Moving along a surface on foot, step by step, so that one foot is always on the ground, such as when strolling, sauntering, walking forwards, backwards or sideways.
Inclusions: walking short or long distances; walking on different surfaces; walking around obstacles
Exclusions: transferring oneself (d420); moving around (d455)

Sources of information:
☒ Case history ☐ Patient-reported questionnaire ☒ Clinical examination ☐ Technical investigation

Description of the problem:
P: *After 30 min. the pain in the leg forces patient to sit or lie down.*
C: *In the VR setting with changing positions patient appears to be slow in walking.*

d455	Moving around	P	0	**1**	2	3	4	8	9
		C	0	1	2	3	4	**8**	9

Moving the whole body from one place to another by means other than walking, such as climbing over a rock or running down a street, skipping, scampering, jumping, somersaulting or running around obstacles.
Inclusions: crawling, climbing, running, jogging, jumping, and swimming
Exclusions: transferring oneself (d420); walking (d450)

Sources of information:
☒ Case history ☐ Patient-reported questionnaire ☒ Clinical examination ☐ Technical investigation

Description of the problem:
P: *Climbing stairs at home several times day is difficult due to pain in the leg.*
C: *No information available*

d720	Complex interpersonal interactions	P	0	**1**	2	3	4	8	9
		C	0	1	2	3	4	**8**	9

Maintaining and managing interactions with other people, in a contextually and socially appropriate manner, such as by regulating emotions and impulses, controlling verbal and physical aggression, acting independently in social interactions and acting in accordance with social rules and conventions.
Inclusions: forming and terminating relationships; regulating behaviours within interactions; interacting according to social rules; and maintaining social space

Sources of information:
☒ Case history ☐ Patient-reported questionnaire ☒ Clinical examination ☐ Technical investigation

Description of the problem:
P: *In interaction with multiple persons, when interrupted in her work, VR counsellors report several problems in emotional impulse control.*
C: *No information available*

Figure 19. Continued on next page

d845	Acquiring, keeping and terminating a job	P	1	2	3	4	8	8	9
		C	1	2	3	4	8	8	9

Seeking, finding and choosing employment, being hired and accepting employment, maintaining and advancing through a job, trade, occupation or profession, and leaving a job in an appropriate manner.
Inclusions: seeking employment; preparing a resume or curriculum vitae; contacting employers and preparing interviews; maintaining a job; monitoring one's own work performance; giving notice; and terminating a job

Sources of information:
☐ Case history ☐ Patient-reported questionnaire ☐ Clinical examination ☐ Technical investigation

Description of the problem:
P: –
C: –

d850	Remunerative employment	P	0	1	2	3	4	8	9
		C	1	2	3	4	8	8	9

Engaging in all aspects of work, as an occupation, trade, profession or other form of employment, for payment, as an employee, full or part time, or self-employed, such as seeking employment and getting a job, doing the required tasks of the job, attending work on time as required, supervising other workers or being supervised, and performing required tasks alone or in groups.
Inclusions: self-employment, part-time and full-time employment

Sources of information:
☒ Case history ☐ Patient-reported questionnaire ☐ Clinical examination ☐ Technical investigation

Description of the problem:
P: Performance of the tasks of her profession as gardener is medically not allowed, therefore not done.
C: –

d855	Non-remunerative employmentb	P	1	2	3	4	8	8	9
		C	1	2	3	4	8	8	9

Engaging in all aspects of work in which pay is not provided, full-time or part-time, including organized work activities, doing the required tasks of the job, attending work on time as required, supervising other workers or being supervised, and performing required tasks alone or in groups, such as volunteer work, charity work, working for a community or religious group without remuneration, working around the home without remuneration.
Exclusion: Chapter 6 Domestic Life

Sources of information:
☐ Case history ☐ Patient-reported questionnaire ☐ Clinical examination ☐ Technical investigation

Description of the problem:
P: –
C: –

Figure 19. Continued on next page

ENVIRONMENTAL FACTORS = make up the physical, social and attitudinal environment in which people live and conduct their lives ***How much of a facilitator or barrier does the person experience with respect to...***		Complete facilitator	Substantial facilitator	Moderate facilitator	Mild facilitator	No barrier/facilitator	Mild barrier	Moderate barrier	Severe barrier	Complete barrier	Not specified	Not applicable
e310	**Immediate family**	+4	+3	**[+2]**	+1	0	**[1]**	2	3	4	8	9
	Individuals related by birth, marriage or other relationship recognized by the culture as immediate family, such as spouses, partners, parents, siblings, children, foster parents, adoptive parents and grandparents. *Exclusions: extended family (e315); personal care providers and personal assistants (e340)*											
	Sources of information: ☒ Case history ☐ Patient-reported questionnaire ☐ Clinical examination ☐ Technical investigation											
	Description of the facilitator/barrier: ***Facilitator:*** *Life partner is supportive for the patient.* ***Barrier:*** *The 12-year-old son has problems in school and with his colleagues and his education takes a lot of energy. This behaviour is reinforced by his father (former husband of the patient).*											
e330	**People in positions of authority**	+4	+3	+2	**[+1]**	0	1	2	3	4	8	9
	Individuals who have decision-making responsibilities for others and who have socially defined influence or power based on their social, economic, cultural or religious roles in society, such as teachers, employers, supervisors, religious leaders, substitute decision-makers, guardians or trustees.											
	Sources of information: ☒ Case history ☐ Patient-reported questionnaire ☐ Clinical examination ☐ Technical investigation											
	Description of the facilitator/barrier: *The former boss of the patient still supports her.*											
e580	**Health services, systems and policies**	+4	+3	**[+2]**	+1	0	**[1]**	2	3	4	8	**[9]**
	Services, systems and policies for preventing and treating health problems, providing medical rehabilitation and promoting a healthy lifestyle. *Exclusion: general social support services, systems and policies (e575)*											
	Sources of information: ☒ Case history ☐ Patient-reported questionnaire ☐ Clinical examination ☐ Technical investigation											
	Description of the facilitator/barrier: ***Facilitator:*** *Directly after accident patient received appropriate treatment.* ***Barrier:*** *Now in the long-term context she feels that there should be a cure or help that is not provided for her.*											

Figure 19. Continued on next page

e590	Labour and employment services, systems and policies	+4	+3	+2	+1	0	1	2	3	4	8	9
	Services, systems and policies related to finding suitable work for persons who are unemployed or looking for different work, or to support individuals already employed who are seeking promotion. *Exclusion: economic services, systems and policies (e565)*											
	Sources of information: ☒ Case history ☐ Patient-reported questionnaire ☐ Clinical examination ☐ Technical investigation											
	Description of the facilitator/barrier: *The labour and employment services provide financial support for the evaluation of new professional possibilities such as the patient's VR rehab program.*											

Figure 19.
ICF Core Set based documentation form based on the ICF Core Set for Vocational Rehabilitation (Brief version)

Note. ICF categories marked in dark grey belong to the Generic Set and are included in any documentation form

* Rating of the nature of the impairment in Body Structures: 0 = no change in structure, 1 = total absence, 2 = partial absence, 3 = additional part, 4 = aberrant dimension, 5 = discontinuity, 6 = deviating position, 7 = qualitative changes in structure, 8 = not specified, 9 = not applicable

** Rating of the location of the impairment in Body Structures: 0 = more than one region, 1 = right, 2 = left, 3 = both sides, 4 = front, 5 = back, 6 = proximal, 7 = distal, 8 = not specified, 9 = not applicable

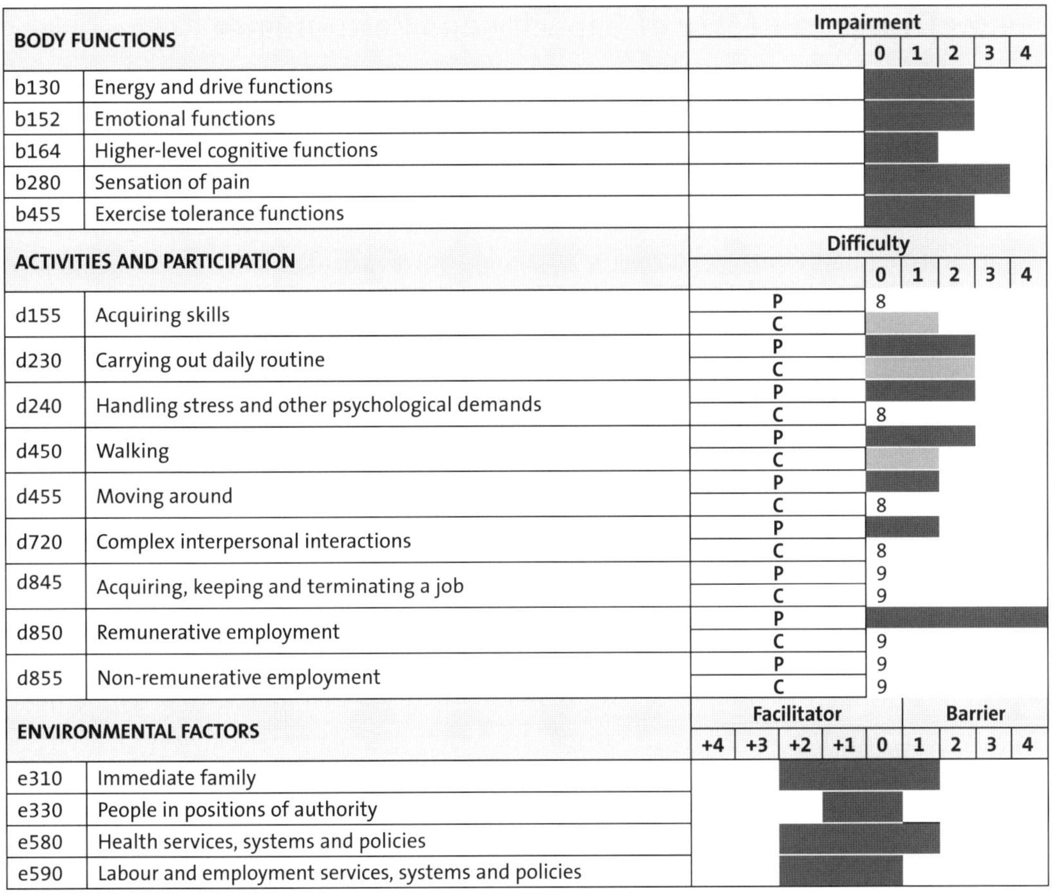

BODY FUNCTIONS		Impairment (0 1 2 3 4)
b130	Energy and drive functions	
b152	Emotional functions	
b164	Higher-level cognitive functions	
b280	Sensation of pain	
b455	Exercise tolerance functions	

ACTIVITIES AND PARTICIPATION			Difficulty (0 1 2 3 4)
d155	Acquiring skills	P	8
		C	
d230	Carrying out daily routine	P	
		C	
d240	Handling stress and other psychological demands	P	
		C	8
d450	Walking	P	
		C	
d455	Moving around	P	
		C	8
d720	Complex interpersonal interactions	P	
		C	8
d845	Acquiring, keeping and terminating a job	P	9
		C	9
d850	Remunerative employment	P	
		C	9
d855	Non-remunerative employment	P	9
		C	9

ENVIRONMENTAL FACTORS		Facilitator (+4 +3 +2 +1) / 0 / Barrier (1 2 3 4)
e310	Immediate family	
e330	People in positions of authority	
e580	Health services, systems and policies	
e590	Labour and employment services, systems and policies	

Figure 20.
Functioning profile of a person following a spine injury and a depressive disorder in a vocational rehabilitation setting

Note. In Body Functions, Body Structures, Activities and Participation: 0 = no problem, 1 = mild problem, 2 = moderate problem, 3 = severe problem, 4 = complete problem; In Environmental Factors: 0 = no barrier/facilitator, 1 = mild barrier, 2 = moderate barrier, 3 = severe barrier, 4 = complete barrier, +1 = mild facilitator, +2 = moderate facilitator, +3 = substantial facilitator, +4 = complete facilitator, 8 = not specified, 9 = not applicable

P = Performance, C = Capacity

5.4.6. Discussion – Use of Capacity and Performance

Mrs. Wilson's case illustrates how crucial it is to evaluate and differentiate between capacity and performance and to decide which information is truly needed for the respective topic and goal. If the information is available, categories should be evaluated in terms of both performance and capacity.

Obtaining reliable information for capacity, however, may be difficult. Capacity evaluation is often very complex and burdensome in time and money or may require technical equipment. Therefore, the use of standardized clinical instruments or tests for capacity evaluation should be carefully chosen and applied. As capacity refers to what the person's intrinsic abilities are and as these are often examined in actual test settings, it is very difficult to assess capacity in an actual workplace where environmental barriers and facilitators may be present.

Capacity plays an essential role in planning interventions directed at improving physical or mental abilities. For chronic conditions where physical or mental changes are not expected, information on performance is more relevant for planning interventions that target work and social reintegration. Information relevant to VR should be collected in situations as close to the real work situation as possible, taking into account the work environment, including adaptations and job challenges over a longer period of time.

In order to gain a comprehensive overview of Mrs. Wilson's functioning, all available and relevant information from different sources was collected to create her functioning profile. The health care professionals in VR situations are vocational counsellors or instructors who often rely on data that they have not evaluated, especially information about physical or cognitive abilities. Capacity evaluation should be performed by the relevant health professional; for example, the physical therapist evaluates the capacity in lifting an object, whereas mental capacities are evaluated by a psychologist.

The description of performance implies the perspective of the client. In a patient-reported questionnaire or in an interview, a patient will usually state his or her performance and not his or her capacity, since capacity is primarily a clinical finding. Performance, as described by the client, is crucial for successful reintegration to the workforce. Moreover, performance information is more reliable than information about his or her capacity in predicting whether the client will actually be able to perform professional activities, because performance takes into account the client's actual work environment.

These differences in evaluating performance and capacity imply that there may be a gap between them. A gap between performance and capacity provides us valuable information about influencing factors of the environment, (called barriers and facilitators in the ICF). In Mrs. Wilson's situation, the focus of VR shifted from enhancing the patient's physical or psychological health in terms of capacity to reintegrating her into the workforce using all environmental support possible. Therefore, new goals were defined in order to find a new profession for her and to enhance her work participation. In this phase of VR, all aspects of strengthening the "performance" are crucial.[83]

In conclusion, this use case shows some of the challenges in assessing performance and assessing capacity and how they can be tackled in order to obtain comprehensive information about the client. Even if the assessment of capacity in a VR setting can prove difficult, both performance and capacity provide important information about the functioning of a client and should be assessed if possible. The comparison between performance and capacity can help identify gaps that allow for a better understanding of the impact of the environment.

5.5. Use Case 5: Applying the ICF Core Set for Low Back Pain in Long-Term Care

Todd Davenport, Sean Rundell and Reuben Escorpizo

This use case illustrates the application of an ICF Core Set for a patient with chronic low back pain (LBP) who attended an outpatient physical therapy clinic. The case demonstrates how highly detailed and technical clinical information gathered in the clinical assessment can be transformed into an ICF-based documentation by means of an ICF Core Set.

5.5.1. The Case

Mrs. Wilkins is a 38-year-old female computer programmer. Her chief concern was a two week history of intermittent right lumbar "burning and pressure" pain. The pain symptom was characterized by a sudden onset when standing after sitting for 3 hours at her computer. She rated her pain as 8/10 at worst, 0/10 at best and 5/10 at the time of her examination. Aggravating activities included sitting two hours or longer, sleeping supine for an hour or longer, jogging longer than 45 minutes and doing activities that involve weight bearing on her right lower extremity. She usually awoke without pain in the morning and experienced pain after sitting at work. Her pain continued to worsen throughout the day. She also reported a secondary concern of burning right lateral leg pain that she experienced intermittently during the last year. This pain began insidiously a year ago, concurrently with multiple brief episodes of LBP. Her episodic LBP resolved, but the leg pain remained, aggravated when jogging or driving or from prolonged sitting.

At the time of intake, she reported that her leg pain increased as her right LBP increased. Her pain eased with changing positions from sitting or supine, using her elliptical machine and using her abdominal exercise equipment. She slept without disturbance when lying on her side. The patient stated that her pain intensity had diminished since initial onset. She reported having no numbness or paresthesia in her lower extremities, change in bowel or bladder function, saddle paresthesia or weakness or incoordination in the lower extremities.

Significant medical history included anxiety disorder and depression. Medications included ibuprofen (600 mg, 3 times daily, as needed) for pain and inflammation, nortriptyline (600 mg, 3 times daily) for depressive symptoms, methylprednisolone (4 mg, once daily) for inflammation, fexofenadine (60 mg, once daily) for allergies and norethindrone (35 mg, once daily) for contraception. Her work activity included sitting at a computer 8 hours a day, and she had a one hour commute to and from work. Her exercise program included jogging, using the elliptical machine and abdominal curls with a floor-exercise apparatus. The patient's goal was to sit 5 hours at work unlimited by pain.

The patient's initial Roland-Morris Disability Questionnaire (RMQ)[84–86] score was 5/24. The RMQ was selected prior to the case due to its sensitivity to change in people with acute LBP.[85] The patient's Fear Avoidance Beliefs Questionnaire (FABQ) scores were 18/42 for the work subscale and 9/24 for the physical activity subscale, indicating low fear-avoidance beliefs.[87] Her Low Back Activity Confidence Scale (LoBACS) scores were 86%, 100% and 90% for the function, self-regulatory and exercise subscales, respectively.[88]

The patient displayed decreased thoracic kyphosis, increased lumbar lordosis and greater prominence of the right lumbar paraspinal musculature with visual postural assessment. Initial pain in a standing position was 1/10 located at the right lumbar spine and lateral leg. During right single-leg stance, the patient had increased lumbar pain and increased pelvic drop with trunk rotation. Left single-leg stance was pain-free with a level pelvis. Myotomal lower-quarter strength screening revealed the L1–L5 innervated muscles were graded as 5/5 and equal bilaterally. The S1 myotome testing demonstrated 8 unilateral heel-raises on the left and 6 unilateral heel-raises on the right, with right heel-raise performance limited by leg pain rather than weakness. Dermatomal light touch was normal. Patellar and Achilles tendon deep tendon reflex tests were 2+ bilaterally. Lumbar active range of motion (AROM) revealed flexion was normal and status quo. Extension was limited with increased right lumbar pain at end-range. Left side bending was limited, and her right lumbar pain was worse at end-range. Right side bending was normal and status quo. Prone hip medial (internal) rotation Passive Range of Motion (PROM) was 56 degrees on the left and 54 degrees on the right, and lateral (external) rotation was 46 degrees on the left and 48 degrees on the right. Straight leg raise was negative with 96 degrees of PROM on the left. Straight leg raise on the right was positive for reproduction of LBP at 88 degrees, and it was unchanged with dorsiflexion sensitizers. Tenderness and restrictions were noted with palpation of the right lumbar paraspinals. The right L5–S1 segment was hypomobile and reproduced her lumbar pain. The left L5–S1 segment was hypomobile and pain-free. The L1–2 through L4–5 segments had normal mobility, which was painful on the right and pain-free on the left.

5.5.2. The Application Area and Setting

The setting was an outpatient physical therapy setting in a closed health system. The typical patient population for this setting consists of individuals seeking secondary or tertiary care for functioning problems or disability related to musculoskeletal pathology.

5.5.3. The Purpose of Applying an ICF Core Set

LBP is among the most common and expensive health conditions in the developed world.[89–93] LBP is also among the most common musculoskeletal conditions treated by physical therapists[94] and a complex biopsychosocial phenomenon. Because of this, a strictly medical approach of pathology and pathophysiology to describe LBP has not led to optimal treatments, both at the population and individual levels. The ICF Core Set provides a useful list of ICF categories that present problems in functioning and its use demonstrates how the ICF Core Set can guide the assessment and evaluation of patient data, which, in turn, can lead to appropriate treatment plans, treatment goals and a better prognosis for the patient.

5.5.4. Selection of the Appropriate ICF Core Set

In general, two steps are required to select an appropriate ICF Core Set. These are the selection of the health condition-related or ICF Core Set related to condition group and the selection of the appropriate type of ICF Core Set (Figure 21).

Choice of ICF Core Set Related to Specific Health Condition or Condition Group

The ICF Core Set for LBP was developed in a long-term care context and hence applies to the current case. Although conflicting evidence exists regarding inter-rater agreement of the ICF Core Set for LBP,[95] evidence generally supports its feasibility for clinical application[96–99] and its content validity.[17, 21–25]

The ICF Core Set for LBP has 78 categories in the Comprehensive version. It includes 19 categories from Body Functions, 5 from Body Structures, 29 from Activities and Participation and 25 from Environmental Factors.[45] The Brief ICF Core Set is a list of 35 essential ICF categories for describing functioning for individuals with LBP.[45]

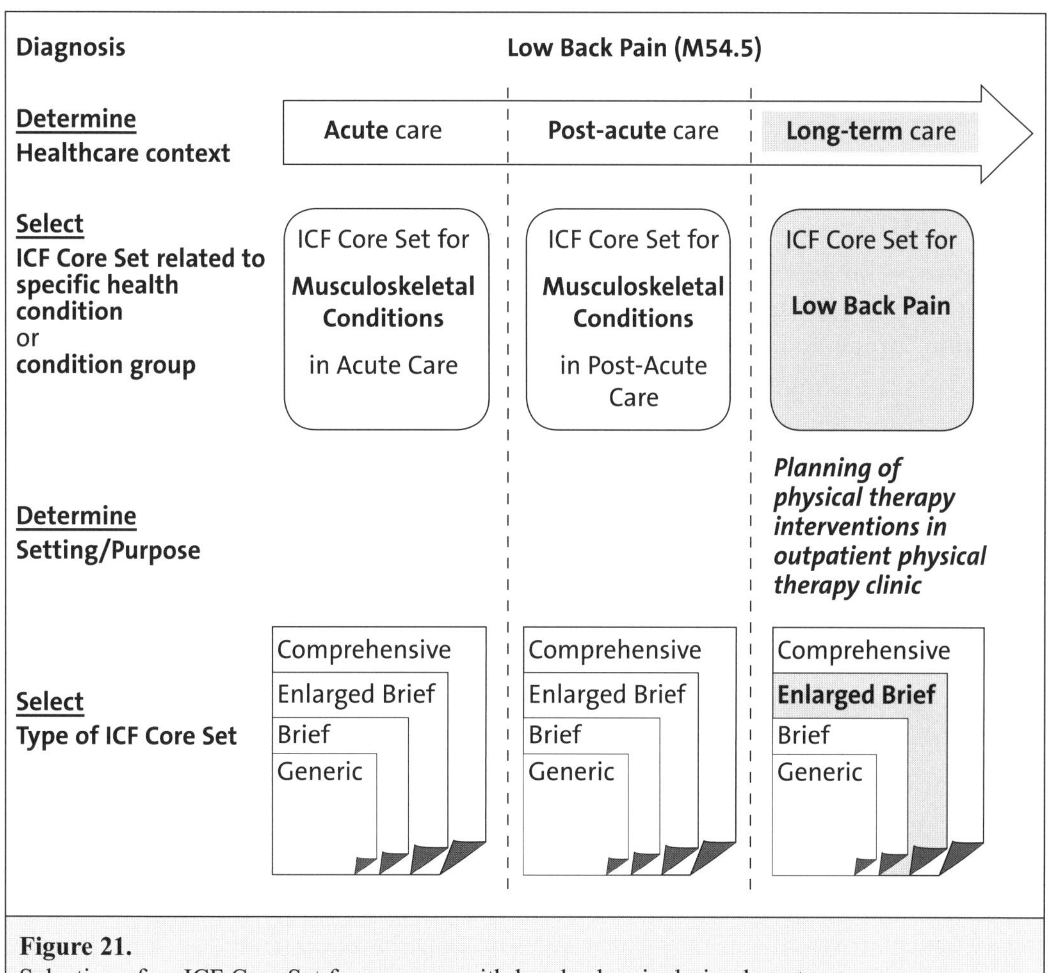

Figure 21.
Selection of an ICF Core Set for a person with low back pain during long-term care

Choice of Type of ICF Core Set

We decided to use the Brief ICF Core Set as the starting point for the description of the patient's level of functioning given the single discipline involved, namely physical therapy. The Brief ICF Core Set for LBP is most useful for many routine clinical applications. As recommended, all of the ICF categories in the Generic Set not already included in the Brief ICF Core Set for LBP have been added. In this case, *d230 Carrying out daily routine* and *d455 Moving around* had to be added. It was also decided to add ICF categories from the Comprehensive ICF Core Set because of the presentation of the patient. As a result, the following categories from the Comprehensive ICF Core Set for LBP were selected: *b265 Touch function*, *b525 Defecation functions*, *b620 Urination functions*, *b750 Motor reflex functions*, *b760*

Control of voluntary movement functions, *d475 Driving* and *d920 Recreation and leisure*. Hence, the result was the Enlarged Brief version.

5.5.5. The Description of Functioning with the Documentation Form

To describe the patient's problems with functioning associated with LBP, the documentation form containing categories from the Generic, the Brief and selected categories from the Comprehensive ICF Core Set for LBP was applied. Information was taken from the patient interview and physical examination, which were designed to cover various areas of patient functioning in ICF domains. Additional objective measurement of the patient's functioning was completed using standardized questionnaires. Selected items from the questionnaires were linked to relevant ICF categories. For example, the RMQ items on house work: "*Because of my back, I am not doing any jobs that I usually do around the house*" and "*I avoid heavy jobs around the house because of my back*" were considered when rating the ICF category *d640 Doing housework*. ICF qualifiers were then used to rate the severity of the patient's functioning problem according to patient interview, questionnaires and physical examination findings. The clinical experience of the physical therapist served as a basis for rating severity to ensure that each finding was interpreted in the context of contemporary physical therapist practice. A global judgment based on the clinician's experience was employed in order to transform scores from standard questionnaires to an ICF qualifier. Each rating was recorded on the documentation form (Figure 22). From this the functioning profile was created (Figure 23). Both figures present the Brief version of the documentation form and the functioning profile (consisting of all ICF categories from the Brief ICF Core Set for LBP with the Generic Set). The full version is available on the CD included with this Manual.

BODY FUNCTIONS = physiological functions of body systems (including psychological functions) ***How much impairment does the person have in...***		No impairment	Mild impairment	Moderate impairment	Severe impairment	Complete impairment	Not specified	Not applicable
b130	**Energy and drive functions**	**0** (selected)	1	2	3	4	8	9
	General mental functions of physiological and psychological mechanisms that cause the individual to move towards satisfying specific needs and general goals in a persistent manner. *Inclusions: functions of energy level, motivation, appetite, craving (including craving for substances that can be abused), and impulse control* *Exclusions: consciousness functions (b110); temperament and personality functions (b126); sleep functions (b134); psychomotor functions (b147); emotional functions (b152)*							
	Sources of information: ☒ Case history ☐ Patient-reported questionnaire ☐ Clinical examination ☐ Technical investigation							
	Description of the problem: *No reported energy and drive impairment.*							
b134	**Sleep functions**	0	1	2	**3** (selected)	4	8	9
	General mental functions of periodic, reversible and selective physical and mental disengagement from one's immediate environment accompanied by characteristic physiological changes. *Inclusions: functions of amount of sleeping, and onset, maintenance and quality of sleep; functions involving the sleep cycle, such as in insomnia, hypersomnia and narcolepsy* *Exclusions: consciousness functions (b110); energy and drive functions (b130); attention functions (b140); psychomotor functions (b147)*							
	Sources of information: ☒ Case history ☒ Patient-reported questionnaire ☐ Clinical examination ☐ Technical investigation							
	Description of the problem: *Activities that aggravate pain included sleeping supine for 1 hour or longer, although the patient awakens without pain in the morning. Roland-Morris Disability Questionnaire indicated that patient "sleeps less well because of her back".*							
b152	**Emotional functions**	**0** (selected)	1	2	3	4	8	9
	Specific mental functions related to the feeling and affective components of the processes of the mind. *Inclusions: functions of appropriateness of emotion, regulation and range of emotion; affect; sadness, happiness, love, fear, anger, hate, tension, anxiety, joy, sorrow; lability of emotion; flattening of affect* *Exclusions: temperament and personality functions (b126); energy and drive functions (b130)*							
	Sources of information: ☒ Case history ☐ Patient-reported questionnaire ☐ Clinical examination ☐ Technical investigation							
	Description of the problem: *Reports depressive symptoms but they are controlled by medication.*							
b280	**Sensation of pain**	0	1	2	**3** (selected)	4	8	9
	Sensation of unpleasant feeling indicating potential or actual damage to some body structure. *Inclusions: sensations of generalized or localized pain in one or more body part, pain in a dermatome, stabbing pain, burning pain, dull pain, aching pain; impairments such as myalgia, analgesia and hyperalgesia*							
	Sources of information: ☒ Case history ☐ Patient-reported questionnaire ☒ Clinical examination ☐ Technical investigation							
	Description of the problem: *Visual Analog Scale (VAS) score indicates severe right lower back pain at worst that limits the patient's activities.*							

Figure 22. Continued on next page

b455	Exercise tolerance functions	■ 0	1	2	3	4	8	9

Functions related to respiratory and cardiovascular capacity as required for enduring physical exertion.
Inclusions: functions of physical endurance, aerobic capacity, stamina and fatigability
Exclusions: functions of the cardiovascular system (b410-b429); haematological system functions (b430); respiration functions (b440); respiratory muscle functions (b445); additional respiratory functions (b450)

Sources of information:
☒ Case history ☐ Patient-reported questionnaire ☐ Clinical examination ☐ Technical investigation

Description of the problem:
No overt impairment of exercise capacity.

b710	Mobility of joint functions	0	1	2	■ 3	4	8	9

Functions of the range and ease of movement of a joint.
Inclusions: functions of mobility of single or several joints, vertebral, shoulder, elbow, wrist, hip, knee, ankle, small joints of hands and feet; mobility of joints generalized; impairments such as in hypermobility of joints, frozen joints, frozen shoulder, arthritis
Exclusions: stability of joint functions (b715); control of voluntary movement functions (b760)

Sources of information:
☐ Case history ☐ Patient-reported questionnaire ☒ Clinical examination ☐ Technical investigation

Description of the problem:
Limited lumbar active range of motion and hip passive range of motion. Hypomobile L5-S1, notably reproducing the symptoms of chief concern on the right side.

b715	Stability of joint functions	■ 0	1	2	3	4	8	9

Functions of the maintenance of structural integrity of the joints.
Inclusions: functions of the stability of a single joint, several joints and joints generalized; impairments such as in unstable shoulder joint, dislocation of a joint, dislocation of shoulder and hip
Exclusion: mobility of joint functions (b710)

Sources of information:
☐ Case history ☐ Patient-reported questionnaire ☒ Clinical examination ☐ Technical investigation

Description of the problem:
Examination findings not indicative of joint instability.

b730	Muscle power functions	0	1	■ 2	3	4	8	9

Functions related to the force generated by the contraction of a muscle or muscle groups.
Inclusions: functions associated with the power of specific muscles and muscle groups, muscles of one limb, one side of the body, the lower half of the body, all limbs, the trunk and the body as a whole; impairments such as weakness of small muscles in feet and hands, muscle paresis, muscle paralysis, monoplegia, hemiplegia, paraplegia, quadriplegia and akinetic mutism
Exclusions: functions of structures adjoining the eye (b215); muscle tone functions (b735); muscle endurance functions (b740)

Sources of information:
☐ Case history ☐ Patient-reported questionnaire ☒ Clinical examination ☐ Technical investigation

Description of the problem:
Gluteal and abdominal weakness indicated by pelvic drop during single leg stance on the right lower extremity. Note, however, that myotomal lower-quarter strength screening revealed the L1-L5 innervated muscles were graded as 5/5 and equal bilaterally

Figure 22. Continued on next page

b735	**Muscle tone functions**	**0** (selected)	1	2	3	4	8	9

Functions related to the tension present in the resting muscles and the resistance offered when trying to move the muscles passively.
Inclusions: functions associated with the tension of isolated muscles and muscle groups, muscles of one limb, one side of the body and the lower half of the body, muscles of all limbs, muscles of the trunk and all muscles of the body; impairments such as hypotonia, hypertonia and muscle spasticity
Exclusions: muscle power functions (b730); muscle endurance functions (b740)

Sources of information:
☐ Case history ☐ Patient-reported questionnaire ☒ Clinical examination ☐ Technical investigation

Description of the problem:
No impairment based on clinical findings

b740	**Muscle endurance functions**	0	1	**2** (selected)	3	4	8	9

Functions related to sustaining muscle contraction for the required period of time.
Functions related to sustaining muscle contraction for the required period of time.
Inclusions: functions associated with sustaining muscle contraction for isolated muscles and muscle groups and all muscles of the body; impairments such as in myasthenia gravis
Exclusions: exercise tolerance functions (b455); muscle power functions (b730); muscle tone functions (b735)

Sources of information:
☐ Case history ☐ Patient-reported questionnaire ☒ Clinical examination ☐ Technical investigation

Description of the problem:
Impairment of gluteal and abdominal muscle endurance indicated by inability to hold level pelvis during right single leg stance.

BODY STRUCTURES = anatomical parts of the body such as organs, limbs and their components ***How much impairment does the person have in the...***		**No impairment**	**Mild impairment**	**Moderate impairment**	**Severe impairment**	**Complete impairment**	**Not specified**	**Not applicable**
s120	**Spinal cord and related structures**	**0** (selected)	1	2	3	4	8	9

Sources of information:
☐ Case history ☐ Patient-reported questionnaire ☒ Clinical examination ☐ Technical investigation

Description of the problem:
Peripheral nervous system examination was normal.

s760	**Structure of trunk**	0	**1** (selected)	2	3	4	8	9

Sources of information:
☐ Case history ☐ Patient-reported questionnaire ☒ Clinical examination ☐ Technical investigation

Description of the problem:
Posture observation revealed mildly thoracic kyphosis and lumbar lordosis..

s770	**Additional musculoskeletal structures related to movement**	0	1	**2** (selected)	3	4	8	9

Sources of information:
☐ Case history ☐ Patient-reported questionnaire ☒ Clinical examination ☐ Technical investigation

Description of the problem:
Straight leg raise on the right was positive for reproduction of low back pain at 88 degrees, and it was unchanged with dorsiflexion sensitizers.

Figure 22. Continued on next page

ACTIVITIES AND PARTICIPATION = execution of a task or action by an individual and involvement in a life situation *How much difficulty does the person have in the...* **P** = *performance of...* **C** = *capacity in...*			No difficulty	Mild difficulty	Moderate difficulty	Severe difficulty	Complete difficulty	Not specified	Not applicable
d230°°	**Carrying out daily routine**	P	**0**	1	2	3	4	8	9
		C	0	1	2	3	4	**8**	9
d240	**Handling stress and other psychological demands**	P	**0**	1	2	3	4	8	9
		C	0	1	2	3	4	**8**	9
d410	**Changing basic body position**	P	0	**1**	2	3	4	8	9
		C	0	**1**	2	3	4	8	9

d230°° Carrying out daily routine

Carrying out simple or complex and coordinated actions in order to plan, manage and complete the requirements of day-to-day procedures or duties, such as budgeting time and making plans for separate activities throughout the day.
Inclusions: managing and completing the daily routine; managing one's own activity level
Exclusion: undertaking multiple tasks (d220)

Sources of information:
☒ Case history ☐ Patient-reported questionnaire ☒ Clinical examination ☐ Technical investigation

Description of the problem:
P: *Patient-reported no limitations*
C: *No information available.*

d240 Handling stress and other psychological demands

Carrying out simple or complex and coordinated actions to manage and control the psychological demands required to carry out tasks demanding significant responsibilities and involving stress, distraction or crises, such as driving a vehicle during heavy traffic or taking care of many children.
Inclusions: handling responsibilities; handling stress and crisis

Sources of information:
☒ Case history ☐ Patient-reported questionnaire ☐ Clinical examination ☐ Technical investigation

Description of the problem:
P: *Patient-reported no significant problem.*
C: *No information available*

d410 Changing basic body position

Getting into and out of a body position and moving from one location to another, such as getting up out of a chair to lie down on a bed, and getting into and out of positions of kneeling or squatting.
Inclusion: changing body position from lying down, from squatting or kneeling, from sitting or standing, bending and shifting the body's centre of gravity
Exclusion: transferring oneself (d420)

Sources of information:
☒ Case history ☒ Patient-reported questionnaire ☒ Clinical examination ☐ Technical investigation

Description of the problem:
P: *Patient-reported no problem with changing body position but that changing position actually eases her lower back pain. Roland-Morris Disability Questionnaire indicated that the patient tries not to bend or kneel down and she lies down to rest more often.*
C: *Patient presents with decreased ability to assume certain lumbar positions and single leg stance on the right lower extremity. .*

Figure 22. Continued on next page

d415	Maintaining a body position	P	0	1	2	**3**	4	8	9
		C	0	**1**	2	3	4	8	9

Staying in the same body position as required, such as remaining seated or remaining standing for work or school.
Inclusions: maintaining a lying, squatting, kneeling, sitting and standing position

Sources of information:
☒ Case history ☐ Patient-reported questionnaire ☒ Clinical examination ☐ Technical investigation

Description of the problem:
***P:** Activities that aggravate pain included maintaining sitting and weight bearing on her right lower extremity.*
***C:** Patient demonstrates mild stance instability on the right lower extremity.*

d410	Changing basic body position	P	0	**1**	2	3	4	8	9
		C	0	1	2	3	**4**	8	9

Getting into and out of a body position and moving from one location to another, such as getting up out of a chair to lie down on a bed, and getting into and out of positions of kneeling or squatting.
Inclusions: changing body position from lying down, from squatting or kneeling, from sitting or standing, bending and shifting the body's centre of gravity
Exclusion: transferring oneself (d420)

Sources of information:
☐ Case history ☐ Patient-reported questionnaire ☒ Clinical examination ☐ Technical investigation

Description of the problem:
***P:** With assistance in sitting up from lying position able to change body position slowly and carefully*
***C:** Without assistance not able (not allowed) to sit up and lay down (due to restrictions related to spinal surgery, problems with shifting the body while sitting due to impaired muscle power and proprioceptive functions*

d430	Lifting and carrying objects	P	**0**	1	2	3	4	8	9
		C	0	1	2	3	4	**8**	9

Raising up an object or taking something from one place to another, such as when lifting a cup or carrying a child from one room to another.
Inclusions: lifting, carrying in the hands or arms, or on shoulders, hip, back or head; putting down

Sources of information:
☒ Case history ☐ Patient-reported questionnaire ☐ Clinical examination ☐ Technical investigation

Description of the problem:
***P:** Patient without self-reported limitation in lifting.*
***C:** No information available*

d450	Walking	P	**0**	1	2	3	4	8	9
		C	**0**	1	2	3	4	8	9

Moving along a surface on foot, step by step, so that one foot is always on the ground, such as when strolling, sauntering, walking forwards, backwards or sideways.
Inclusions: walking short or long distances; walking on different surfaces; walking around obstacles
Exclusions: transferring oneself (d420); moving around (d455)

Sources of information:
☒ Case history ☐ Patient-reported questionnaire ☒ Clinical examination ☐ Technical investigation

Description of the problem:
***P:** Patient reports being able to walk independently without limitation;*
***C:** No significant finding based on clinical examination (direct observation).*

Figure 22. Continued on next page

d455[∞]	**Moving around**	P	**0**	1	2	3	4	8	9
		C	0	1	2	3	4	**8**	9

Moving the whole body from one place to another by means other than walking, such as climbing over a rock or running down a street, skipping, scampering, jumping, somersaulting or running around obstacles.
Inclusions: crawling, climbing, running, jogging, jumping, and swimming
Exclusions: transferring oneself (d420); walking (d450)

Sources of information:
☒ Case history ☐ Patient-reported questionnaire ☐ Clinical examination ☐ Technical investigation

Description of the problem:
P: *Patient moves around independently without limitation.*
C: *No information available*

d530	**Toileting**	P	**0**	1	2	3	4	8	9
		C	0	1	2	3	4	**8**	9

Planning and carrying out the elimination of human waste (menstruation, urination and defecation) and cleaning oneself afterwards.
Inclusions: regulating urination, defecation and menstrual care
Exclusions: washing oneself (d510); caring for body parts (d520)

Sources of information:
☒ Case history ☐ Patient-reported questionnaire ☐ Clinical examination ☐ Technical investigation

Description of the problem:
P: *No limitation reported from the patient; does not need any devices or assistance*
C: *No information available*

d540	**Dressing**	P	**0**	1	2	3	4	8	9
		C	0	1	2	3	4	**8**	9

Carrying out the coordinated actions and tasks of putting on and taking off clothes and footwear in sequence and in keeping with climatic and social conditions, such as by putting on, adjusting and removing shirts, skirts, blouses, pants, undergarments, saris, kimono, tights, hats, gloves, coats, shoes, boots, sandals and slippers.
Inclusions: putting on or taking off clothes and footwear and choosing appropriate clothing

Sources of information:
☒ Case history ☐ Patient-reported questionnaire ☐ Clinical examination ☐ Technical investigation

Description of the problem:
P: *No limitation reported from the patient; does not need any devices or assistance*
C: *No information available*

Figure 22. Continued on next page

d640	**Doing housework**	P	0	1	**2**	3	4	8	9
		C	0	1	2	3	4	**8**	9

Managing a household by cleaning the house, washing clothes, using household appliances, storing food and disposing of garbage, such as by sweeping, mopping, washing counters, walls and other surfaces; collecting and disposing of household garbage; tidying rooms, closets and drawers; collecting, washing, drying, folding and ironing clothes; cleaning footwear; using brooms, brushes and vacuum cleaners; using washing machines, driers and irons.
Inclusions: washing and drying clothes and garments; cleaning cooking area and utensils; cleaning living area; using household appliances, storing daily necessities and disposing of garbage
Exclusions: acquiring a place to live (d610); acquisition of goods and services (d620); preparing meals (d630); caring for household objects (d650); caring for others (d660)

Sources of information:

☐ Case history ☒ Patient-reported questionnaire ☐ Clinical examination ☐ Technical investigation

Description of the problem:

P: *Roland-Morris Disability Questionnaire indicated "avoiding heavy jobs around the house because of her back" and "not doing any jobs that she usually does around the house".*
C: *No information available*

d415	**Family relationships**	P	**0**	1	2	3	4	8	9
		C	0	1	2	3	4	**8**	9

Creating and maintaining kinship relationships, such as with members of the nuclear family, extended family, foster and adopted family and step-relationships, more distant relationships such as second cousins or legal guardians.
Inclusions: parent-child and child-parent relationships, sibling and extended family relationships

Sources of information:

☒ Case history ☐ Patient-reported questionnaire ☒ Clinical examination ☐ Technical investigation

Description of the problem:

P: *No restriction reported in family functioning*
C: *No information available*

d845	**Acquiring, keeping and terminating and job**	P	0	1	2	3	4	8	**9**
		C	0	1	2	3	4	8	**9**

Seeking, finding and choosing employment, being hired and accepting employment, maintaining and advancing through a job, trade, occupation or profession, and leaving a job in an appropriate manner.

Inclusions: seeking employment; preparing a resume or curriculum vitae; contacting employers and preparing interviews; maintaining a job; monitoring one's own work performance; giving notice; and terminating a job

Sources of information:

☒ Case history ☐ Patient-reported questionnaire ☐ Clinical examination ☐ Technical investigation

Description of the problem:

P: –
C: –

Figure 22. Continued on next page

d850	Remunerative employment	P	0	1	2	**3**	4	8	9
		C	0	1	2	3	4	**8**	9

Engaging in all aspects of work, as an occupation, trade, profession or other form of employment, for payment, as an employee, full or part time, or self-employed, such as seeking employment and getting a job, doing the required tasks of the job, attending work on time as required, supervising other workers or being supervised, and performing required tasks alone or in groups.
Inclusions: self-employment, part-time and full-time employment

Sources of information:
☒ Case history ☐ Patient-reported questionnaire ☐ Clinical examination ☐ Technical investigation

Description of the problem:
P: *Patient is unable to sit according to work requirements.*
C: *No information available*

d859	Work and employment, specified and other unspecified	P	0	1	2	3	4	8	**9**
		C	0	1	2	3	4	8	**9**

Engaging in any form of play, recreational or leisure activity, such as informal or organized play and sports, programmes of physical fitness, relaxation, amusement or diversion, going to art galleries, museums, cinemas or theatres; engaging in crafts or hobbies, reading for enjoyment, playing musical instruments; sightseeing, tourism and travelling for pleasure.
Inclusions: play, sports, arts and culture, crafts, hobbies and socializing

Sources of information:
☒ Case history ☐ Patient-reported questionnaire ☐ Clinical examination ☐ Technical investigation

Description of the problem:
P: –
C: –

ENVIRONMENTAL FACTORS
= make up the physical, social and attitudinal environment in which people live and conduct their lives

How much of a facilitator or barrier does the person experience with respect to...

		Complete facilitator	Substantial facilitator	Moderate facilitator	Mild facilitator	No barrier/facilitator	Mild barrier	Moderate barrier	Substantial barrier	Complete barrier	Not specified	Not applicable
e110	Products or substances for personal consumption	**+4**	+3	+2	+1	0	1	2	3	4	8	9

Any natural or human-made object or substance gathered, processed or manufactured for ingestion.
Inclusions: food, drink and drugs

Sources of information:
☒ Case history ☐ Patient-reported questionnaire ☐ Clinical examination ☐ Technical investigation

Description of the facilitator/barrier:
Receives medication appropriate for her condition.

Figure 22. Continued on next page

e135	Products and technology for employment	+4	+3	+2	+1	0	1	**2**	3	4	8	9

Equipment, products and technologies used by people in daily activities, including those adapted or specially designed, located in, on or near the person using them.
Inclusions: general and assistive products and technology for personal use

Sources of information:
☒ Case history ☐ Patient-reported questionnaire ☐ Clinical examination ☐ Technical investigation

Description of the facilitator/barrier:
Current workplace ergonomics are suboptimal secondary to contribute to pain while sitting for work requirements.

e155	Design, construction and building products and technology of buildings for private use	+4	+3	+2	+1	**0**	1	2	3	4	8	9

Products and technology that constitute an individual's indoor and outdoor human-made environment that is planned, designed and constructed for private use, including those adapted or specially designed.
Inclusions: design, construction and building products and technology of entrances and exits, facilities and routing

Sources of information:
☒ Case history ☐ Patient-reported questionnaire ☐ Clinical examination ☐ Technical investigation

Description of the facilitator/barrier:
No self reported deficits in functioning related to non-work functions; aspects of current exercise regime that involve equipment are reported to temporarily ease symptoms. No self-reported impact

e310	Immediate family	+4	+3	+2	+1	**0**	1	2	3	4	8	9

Individuals related by birth, marriage or other relationship recognized by the culture as immediate family, such as spouses, partners, parents, siblings, children, foster parents, adoptive parents and grandparents.
Exclusions: extended family (e315); personal care providers and personal assistants (e340)

Sources of information:
☒ Case history ☐ Patient-reported questionnaire ☐ Clinical examination ☐ Technical investigation

Description of the facilitator/barrier:
No self-reported impact of functioning based on immediate family relationships

e355	Health professionals	**+4**	+3	+2	+1	0	1	2	3	4	8	9

All service providers working within the context of the health system, such as doctors, nurses, physiotherapists, occupational therapists, speech therapists, audiologists, orthotist-prosthetists, medical social workers.
Exclusion: other professionals (e360)

Sources of information:
☒ Case history ☐ Patient-reported questionnaire ☐ Clinical examination ☐ Technical investigation

Description of the facilitator/barrier:
Receives support from medical doctor, nurse and physical therapist

Figure 22. Continued on next page

e410	**Individual attitudes of immediate family members**	+4	+3	+2	+1	0	1	2	3	4	**8**	9
	General or specific opinions and beliefs of immediate family members about the person or about other matters (e.g. social, political and economic issues) that influence individual behaviour and actions.											
	Sources of information: ☒ Case history ☐ Patient-reported questionnaire ☐ Clinical examination ☐ Technical investigation											
	Description of the facilitator/barrier: *Not specifically assessed secondary to family not commonly available in this practice setting*											
e450	**Individual attitudes of health professionals**	+4	**+3**	+2	+1	0	1	2	3	4	8	9
	General or specific opinions and beliefs of health professionals about the person or about other matters (e.g. social, political and economic issues) that influence individual behaviour and actions.											
	Sources of information: ☒ Case history ☐ Patient-reported questionnaire ☐ Clinical examination ☐ Technical investigation											
	Description of the facilitator/barrier: *Experiences health professionals as very supportive, although she is impatient with current clinical management secondary to lack of improvement prior to starting physical therapy*											
e550	**Legal services, systems and policies**	+4	+3	+2	+1	**0**	1	2	3	4	8	9
	Services, systems and policies concerning the legislation and other law of a country.											
	Sources of information: ☒ Case history ☐ Patient-reported questionnaire ☐ Clinical examination ☐ Technical investigation											
	Description of the facilitator/barrier: *No barrier or facilitator was identified*											
e570	**Social security services, systems and policies**	+4	+3	+2	+1	**0**	1	2	3	4	8	9
	Services, systems and policies aimed at providing income support to people who, because of age, poverty, unemployment, health condition or disability, require public assistance that is funded either by general tax revenues or contributory schemes.											
	Sources of information: ☒ Case history ☐ Patient-reported questionnaire ☐ Clinical examination ☐ Technical investigation											
	Description of the facilitator/barrier: *No barrier or facilitator was identified*											

Figure 22. Continued on next page

e580	Health services, systems and policies	**+4**	+3	+2	+1	0	1	2	3	4	8	9
	Services, systems and policies for preventing and treating health problems, providing medical rehabilitation and promoting a healthy lifestyle. *Exclusion: general social support services, systems and policies (e575)*											
	Sources of information: ☒ Case history ☐ Patient-reported questionnaire ☐ Clinical examination ☐ Technical investigation											
	Description of the facilitator/barrier: *Treatment is being paid completely by her health insurance without co-payment or additional premiums*											

Figure 22.
ICF Core Set based documentation form based on the ICF Core Set for Low Back Pain (Brief version)

Note. ICF categories marked in dark grey belong to the Generic Set and are included in any documentation form

∞ Category from the Generic Set not included in the ICF Core Set for Low Back Pain

* Rating of the nature of the impairment in Body Structures: 0 = no change in structure, 1 = total absence, 2 = partial absence, 3 = additional part, 4 = aberrant dimension, 5 = discontinuity, 6 = deviating position, 7 = qualitative changes in structure, 8 = not specified, 9 = not applicable

** Rating of the location of the impairment in Body Structures: 0 = more than one region, 1 = right, 2 = left, 3 = both sides, 4 = front, 5 = back, 6 = proximal, 7 = distal, 8 = not specified, 9 = not applicable

BODY FUNCTIONS			Impairment				
			0	1	2	3	4
b130	Energy and drive functions						
b134	Sleep functions						
b152	Emotional functions						
b280	Sensation of pain						
b455	Exercise tolerance functions						
b710	Mobility of joint functions						
b715	Stability of joint functions						
b730	Muscle power functions						
b735	Muscle tone functions						
b740	Muscle endurance functions						
BODY STRUCTURES			**Impairment**				
			0	1	2	3	4
s120	Spinal cord and related structures						
s760	Structure of trunk						
s770	Additional musculoskeletal structures related to movement						

ACTIVITIES AND PARTICIPATION			Difficulty 0	1	2	3	4
d230∞	Carrying out daily routine	P					
		C	8				
d240	Handling stress and other psychological demands	P					
		C	8				
d410	Changing basic body position	P					
		C					
d415	Maintaining a body position	P					
		C					
d430	Lifting and carrying objects	P					
		C	8				
d450	Walking	P					
		C					
d455∞	Moving around	P					
		C	8				
d530	Toileting	P					
		C	8				
d540	Dressing	P					
		C	8				
d640	Doing housework	P					
		C	8				
d760	Family relationships	P					
		C	8				
d845	Acquiring, keeping and terminating and job	P	9				
		C	9				
d850	Remunerative employment	P					
		C	8				
d859	Work and employment, specified and other unspecified	P	9				
		C	9				

ENVIRONMENTAL FACTORS		Facilitator +4	+3	+2	+1	0	Barrier 1	2	3	4
e110	Products or substances for personal consumption									
e135	Products and technology for employment									
e155	Design, construction, building products and technology of buildings, private use									
e310	Immediate family									
e355	Health professionals									
e410	Individual attitudes of immediate family members					8				
e450	Individual attitudes of health-related professionals									
e550	Legal services, systems and policies									
e570	Social security services, systems and policies									
e580	Health services, systems and policies									

Figure 23.
Functioning profile of a person with low back pain (Brief version)

Note. In Body Functions, Body Structures, Activities and Participation: 0 = no problem, 1 = mild problem, 2 = moderate problem, 3 = severe problem, 4 = complete problem; In Environmental Factors: 0 = no barrier/facilitator, 1 = mild barrier, 2 = moderate barrier, 3 = severe barrier, 4 = complete barrier, +1 = mild facilitator, +2 = moderate facilitator, +3 = substantial facilitator, +4 = complete facilitator, 8 = not specified, 9 = not applicable

P = Performance, C = Capacity

∞ ICF category from the Generic Set not included in the ICF Core Set for Low Back Pain

5.5.6. Discussion – Representing Detailed Clinical Information Using an ICF Core Set

The ICF Core Set for LBP appears to provide an effective framework for physical therapists to better understand each person's experience with his or her functioning problems associated with LBP. In this case, a variety of existing valid and reliable clinical assessments (patient- or clinician-reported) were utilized to assess the various domains of functioning that are commonly assessed in the outpatient physical therapy setting. Thus, this case demonstrates the transformation of detailed clinical information to an ICF Core Set-based documentation. The ICF Core Set for LBP was valuable in the transformation process without foregoing the vital information from the standard sources (i.e. case history, standard questionnaires, and clinical and technical examinations). The ICF Core Set facilitated the organization of examination findings which were transformed to the ICF categories and ICF qualifiers, resulting in an ICF-based functioning profile of the patient.

The ICF Core Set for LBP helped to identify impairments of Body Structure and Body Function and Activity limitations and Participation restrictions and the impact of Environmental Factors. Interventions directed at these impairments, limitations and restrictions, and relevant contextual factors can address the impact of the health condition and helped to affect the Activities and Participation of the patient. For example, the painful hypomobility of the lumbar spine played a great role in the patient's functioning since it contributed to the restrictions in work participation.

There are four points that need to be kept in mind with this use case. First, while detailed clinical information from case histories or medical records is often in separate documents that are differently structured, the ICF Core Set-based documentation form unifies this information and enables users to easily locate specific information. For example, to search for particular clinical information in the case history provided in the first part of this use case, the user would have to go through the entire case history to find the patient's list of medication. In contrast, this information can easily be found in the ICF category *e1101 Drugs* of the ICF Core Set-based documentation form. Secondly, in this case, detailed clinical information may be too comprehensive, with technical information only relevant to examinations in physical therapy. The advantage of transforming this information to an ICF Core Set documentation form, however, is that it aggregates the specific information in a manner that is understandable to other health professionals. Thirdly, users always have the option of adding relevant ICF categories to the Brief ICF Core Set from the Comprehensive ICF Core Set or the whole ICF, if necessary. In this case, *b620 Urination functions*, *b750 Motor reflex functions*, *d475 Driving* and *d920 Recreation and leisure* from the Comprehensive ICF Core Set for LBP were all added as they are relevant to this case.

Finally, while linking areas examined during patient assessment to an ICF category is an easy matter, transforming an existing measurement scale to the ICF qualifiers can be challenging. For instance, the RMQ is not clear how it defines varying levels of disability and presents this as a checklist rather than as a scale. Pending futher research in this area, the selection of an equivalent ICF qualifier depends heavily on the experience of the physical therapist with the health condition, as well as their experience with the particular outcome measure being used, since the transformation of a standard scale to an ICF qualifier does not necessarily mean a one-to-one conversion.

In conclusion, this use case illustrates the selection process of the ICF Core Set for a person with LBP. This selection resulted in an ICF-based description of the patient's overall functioning and specific areas of functioning attributed to LBP. Moreover, we were able to transform the information obtained from standard measures, patient-reported questionaires and clinical examination procedures, typically administered in an outpatient physical therapy clinical setting, to the ICF. In turn, the organisation and evaluation of examination findings according to the ICF Core Set for LBP aided us in determining and prioritising optimal interventions, as well as identifying key outcomes measures.

Acknowledgement

Portions of this chapter were excerpted and with some modification from *Rundell SD, Davenport TE, Wagner TW (2009).* Physical therapist management of acute and chronic low back pain using the World Health Organization's International Classification of Functioning, Disability and Health. *Physical Therapy, 89(1):82–90,* with kind permission of the American Physical Therapy Association.

6 References

1. Ustun B, Chatterji S, Kostanjsek N. Comments from WHO for the Journal of Rehabilitation Medicine Special Supplement on ICF Core Sets. J Rehabil Med 2004;44S:7–8.
2. Stucki G, Ustun TB, Melvin J. Applying the ICF for the acute hospital and early post-acute rehabilitation facilities. Disabil Rehabil 2005;27:349–52.
3. Callahan D. The WHO definition of "health". Stud Hastings Cent 1973;1:77–88.
4. Stucki G, Cieza A, Melvin J. The International Classification of Functioning, Disability and Health (ICF): a unifying model for the conceptual description of the rehabilitation strategy. J Rehabil Med 2007;39:279–85.
5. Stucki G, Boonen A, Tugwell P, Cieza A, Boers M. The World Health Organisation International Classification of Functioning, Disability and Health: a conceptual model and interface for the OMERACT process. J Rheumatol 2007;34:600–66.
6. WHO. International Classification of Functioning, Disability and Health. Geneva: World Health Organization; 2001.
7. Madden R, Sykes C, Ustun B, World Health Organization Family of International Classifications: Definition, scope and purpose. Available at http://www.who.int/classifications/en/FamilyDocument2007.pdf.
8. WHO. International Statistical Classification of Diseases and Related Health Problems, Tenth Revision, Vols. 1–3. Geneva: World Health Organisation; 1992–1994.
9. Cieza A, Stucki G. New approaches to understanding the impact of musculoskeletal conditions. Best Pract Res Clin Rheumatol 2004;18:141–54.
10. Stucki G, Kostanjsek N, Ustun B, Cieza A. ICF-based classification and measurement of functioning. Eur J Phys Rehabil Med 2008;44:315–28.
11. Stucki G, Grimby G. Applying the ICF in medicine. J Rehabil Med 2004;44S:5–6.
12. Kostanjsek N, Rubinelli S, Escorpizo R, Cieza A, Kennedy C, Selb M, Stucki G, Ustun TB. Assessing the impact of health conditions using the ICF. Disabil Rehabil 2011;33:1475–82.

13. Stucki G, Cieza A, Ewert T, Kostanjsek N, Chatterji S, Ustun TB. Application of the International Classification of Functioning, Disability and Health (ICF) in clinical practice. Disabil Rehabil 2002;24:281–82.

14. Ewert T, Fuessl M, Cieza A, Andersen C, Chatterji S, Kostanjsek N, Stucki G. Identification of the most common patient problems in patients with chronic conditions using the ICF checklist. J Rehabil Med 2004;44S:22–9.

15. Weigl M, Cieza A, Andersen C, Kollerits B, Amann E, Stucki G. Identification of relevant ICF categories in patients with chronic health conditions: a Delphi exercise. J Rehabil Med 2004;44S:12–21.

16. Brockow T, Wohlfahrt K, Hillert A, Geyh S, Weigl M, Franke T, Resch KL, Cieza A. Identifying the concepts contained in outcome measures of clinical trials on depressive disorders using the International Classification of Functioning, Disability and Health as a reference. J Rehabil Med 2004;44S:49–55.

17. Brockow T, Duddeck K, Geyh S, Schwarzkopf S, Weigl M, Franke T, Brach M. Identifying the concepts contained in outcome measures of clinical trials on breast cancer using the International Classification of Functioning, Disability and Health as a reference. J Rehabil Med 2004;44S:43–8.

18. Brockow T, Cieza A, Kuhlow H, Sigl T, Franke T, Harder M, Stucki G. Identifying the concepts contained in outcome measures of clinical trials on musculoskeletal disorders and chronic widespread pain using the International Classification of Functioning, Disability and Health as a reference. J Rehabil Med 2004;44S:30–6.

19. Wolff B, Cieza A, Parentin A, Rauch A, Sigl T, Brockow T, Stucki A. Identifying the concepts contained in outcome measures of clinical trials on four internal disorders using the International Classification of Functioning, Disability and Health as a reference. J Rehabil Med 2004;44S:37–42.

20. Geyh S, Kurt T, Brockow T, Cieza A, Ewert T, Omar Z, Resch KL. Identifying the concepts contained in outcome measures of clinical trials on stroke using the International Classification of Functioning, Disability and Health as a reference. J Rehabil Med 2004;44S:56–62.

21. Grill E, Stucki G. Criteria for validating comprehensive ICF Core Sets and developing brief ICF Core Set versions. J Rehabil Med 2011;43:87–91.

22. Kirchberger I, Coenen M, Hierl FX, Dieterle C, Seissler J, Stucki G, Cieza A. Validation of the International Classification of Functioning, Disability and Health (ICF) core set for diabetes mellitus from the patient perspective using focus groups. Diabet Med 2009;26:700–7.

23. Coenen M, Cieza A, Stamm TA, Amann E, Kollerits B, Stucki G. Validation of the International Classification of Functioning, Disability and Health (ICF) Core Set for rheumatoid arthritis from the patient perspective using focus groups. Arthritis Res Ther 2006;8(4):R84.

24. Stamm TA, Cieza A, Coenen M, Machold KP, Nell VP, Smolen JS, Stucki G. Validating the International Classification of Functioning, Disability and Health Comprehensive Core Set for Rheumatoid Arthritis from the patient perspective: a qualitative study. Arthritis Rheum 2005;53:431–9.

25. Cieza A, Ewert T, Ustun TB, Chatterji S, Kostanjsek N, Stucki G. Development of ICF Core Sets for patients with chronic conditions. J Rehabil Med 2004;44S:9–11.

26. ICF Research Branch. Available at www.icf-research-branch.org/icf-core-sets-projects.html. Last accessed July 2011

27. Ewert T, Grill E, Bartholomeyczik S, Finger M, Mokrusch T, Kostanjsek N, Stucki G. ICF Core Set for patients with neurological conditions in the acute hospital. Disabil Rehabil 2005;27:367–73.

28. Grill E, Ewert T, Chatterji S, Kostanjsek N, Stucki G. ICF Core Sets development for the acute hospital and early post-acute rehabilitation facilities. Disabil Rehabil 2005;27:361–66.

29. Stier-Jarmer M, Grill E, Ewert T, Bartholomeyczik S, Finger M, Mokrusch T, Kostanjsek N, Stucki G. ICF Core Set for patients with neurological conditions in early post-acute rehabilitation facilities. Disabil Rehabil 2005;27:389–95.

30. Coenen M, Cieza A, Freeman J, Khan F, Miller D, Weise A, Kesselring J. The development of ICF Core Sets for multiple sclerosis: results of the International Consensus Conference. J Neurol 2011;258(8):1477–88.

31. Geyh S, Cieza A, Schouten J, Dickson H, Frommelt P, Omar Z, Kostanjsek N, Ring H, Stucki G. ICF Core Sets for stroke. J Rehabil Med 2004:135–41.

32. Bernabeu M, Laxe S, Lopez R, Stucki G, Ward A, Barnes M, Kostanjsek N, Reed G, Tate R, Whyte J, Zasler N, Cieza A. Developing core sets for persons with traumatic brain injury based on the International Classification of Functioning, Disability and Health. Neurorehabil Neural Repair 2009;23:464–67.

33. Kirchberger I, Cieza A, Biering-Sorensen F, Baumberger M, Charlifue S, Post MW, Campbell R, Kovindha A, Ring H, Sinnott A, Kostanjsek N, Stucki G. ICF Core Sets for individuals with spinal cord injury in the early post-acute context. Spinal Cord 2010;48:297–304.

34. Cieza A, Kirchberger I, Biering-Sorensen F, Baumberger M, Charlifue S, Post MW, Campbell R, Kovindha A, Ring H, Sinnott A, Kostanjsek N, Stucki G. ICF Core Sets for individuals with spinal cord injury in the long-term context. Spinal Cord 2010;48:305–12.

35. Boldt C, Grill E, Wildner M, Portenier L, Wilke S, Stucki G, Kostanjsek N, Quittan M. ICF Core Set for patients with cardiopulmonary conditions in the acute hospital. Disabil Rehabil 2005;27:375–80.

36. Wildner M, Quittan M, Portenier L, Wilke S, Boldt C, Stucki G, Kostanjsek N, Grill E. ICF Core Set for patients with cardiopulmonary conditions in early post-acute rehabilitation facilities. Disabil Rehabil 2005;27:397–404.

37. Cieza A, Stucki A, Geyh S, Berteanu M, Quittan M, Simon A, Kostanjsek N, Stucki G, Walsh N. ICF Core Sets for chronic ischaemic heart disease. J Rehabil Med 2004;44S:94–9.

38. Ruof J, Cieza A, Wolff B, Angst F, Ergeletzis D, Omar Z, Kostanjsek N, Stucki G. ICF Core Sets for diabetes mellitus. J Rehabil Med 2004;44S:100–6.

39. Stucki A, Daansen P, Fuessl M, Cieza A, Huber E, Atkinson R, Kostanjsek N, Stucki G, Ruof J. ICF Core Sets for obesity. J Rehabil Med 2004;44S:107–13.

40. Stucki A, Stoll T, Cieza A, Weigl M, Giardini A, Wever D, Kostanjsek N, Stucki G. ICF Core Sets for obstructive pulmonary diseases. J Rehabil Med 2004;44S:114–20.

41. Stoll T, Brach M, Huber EO, Scheuringer M, Schwarzkopf SR, Konstanjsek N, Stucki G. ICF Core Set for patients with musculoskeletal conditions in the acute hospital. Disabil Rehabil 2005;27:381–7.

42. Scheuringer M, Stucki G, Huber EO, Brach M, Schwarzkopf SR, Kostanjsek N, Stoll T. ICF Core Set for patients with musculoskeletal conditions in early post-acute rehabilitation facilities. Disabil Rehabil 2005;27:405–10.

43. Boonen A, Braun J, van der Horst Bruinsma IE, Huang F, Maksymowych W, Kostanjsek N, Cieza A, Stucki G, van der Heijde D. ASAS/WHO ICF Core Sets for ankylosing spondylitis (AS): how to classify the impact of AS on functioning and health. Ann Rheum Dis 2010;69:102–7.

44. Cieza A, Stucki G, Weigl M, Kullmann L, Stoll T, Kamen L, Kostanjsek N, Walsh N. ICF Core Sets for chronic widespread pain. J Rehabil Med 2004;44S:63–8.

45. Cieza A, Stucki G, Weigl M, Disler P, Jackel W, van der Linden S, Kostanjsek N, de Bie R. ICF Core Sets for low back pain. J Rehabil Med 2004;44S:69–74.

46. Dreinhofer K, Stucki G, Ewert T, Huber E, Ebenbichler G, Gutenbrunner C, Kostanjsek N, Cieza A. ICF Core Sets for osteoarthritis. J Rehabil Med 2004;44S:75–80.

47. Cieza A, Schwarzkopf S, Sigl T, Stucki G, Melvin J, Stoll T, Woolf A, Kostanjsek N, Walsh N. ICF Core Sets for osteoporosis. J Rehabil Med 2004;44S:81–6.

48. Stucki G, Cieza A, Geyh S, Battistella L, Lloyd J, Symmons D, Kostanjsek N, Schouten J. ICF Core Sets for rheumatoid arthritis. J Rehabil Med 2004;44S:87–93.

49. Grill E, Zochling J, Stucki G, Mittrach R, Scheuringer M, Liman W, Kostanjsek N, Braun J. International Classification of Functioning, Disability and Health (ICF) Core Set for patients with acute arthritis. Clin Exp Rheumatol 2007;25:252–58.

50. Grill E, Hermes R, Swoboda W, Uzarewicz C, Kostanjsek N, Stucki G. ICF Core Set for geriatric patients in early post-acute rehabilitation facilities. Disabil Rehabil 2005;27:411–17.

51. Vieta E, Cieza A, Stucki G, Chatterji S, Nieto M, Sanchez-Moreno J, Jaeger J, Grunze H, Ayuso-Mateos JL. Developing core sets for persons with bipolar disorder based on the International Classification of Functioning, Disability and Health. Bipolar Disord 2007;9:16–24.

52. Cieza A, Chatterji S, Andersen C, Cantista P, Herceg M, Melvin J, Stucki G, de Bie R. ICF Core Sets for depression. J Rehabil Med 2004;44S:128–34.

53. Brach M, Cieza A, Stucki G, Fussl M, Cole A, Ellerin B, Fialka-Moser V, Kostanjsek N, Melvin J. ICF Core Sets for breast cancer. J Rehabil Med 2004;44S:121–27.

54. Tschiesner U, Rogers S, Dietz A, Yueh B, Cieza A. Development of ICF core sets for head and neck cancer. Head Neck 2010;32:210–20.

55. Rudolf KD, Kus S, Chung KC, Johnston M, LeBlanc M, Cieza A. Development of the International Classification of Functioning, Disability and Health Core Sets for hand conditions: results of the World Health Organization international consensus process. Disabil & Rehabil 2012;34(8):681–93.

56. Peyrin-Biroulet L, Cieza A, Sandborn WJ, Kostanjsek N, Kamm MA, Hibi T, Lemann M, Stucki G, Colombel JF. Disability in inflammatory bowel diseases: developing ICF Core Sets for patients with inflammatory bowel diseases based on the International Classification of Functioning, Disability and Health. Inflamm Bowel Dis 2010;16:15–22.

57. Gradinger F, Cieza A, Stucki A, Michel F, Bentley A, Oksenberg A, Rogers AE, Stucki G, Partinen M. Part 1. International Classification of Functioning, Disability and Health (ICF) Core Sets for persons with sleep disorders: results of the consensus process integrating evidence from preparatory studies. Sleep Med 2011;12:92–6.

58. Finger ME, Escorpizo R, Glässel A, Gmünder HP, Lückenkemper M, Chan C, Fritz J, Studer U, Ekholm J, Kostanjsek N, Stucki G, Cieza A. ICF Core Set for vocational rehabilitation: results of an international consensus conference. Disabil Rehabil 2012;34(5):429–38.

59. Grill E, Quittan M, Fialka-Moser V, Muller M, Strobl R, Kostanjsek N, Stucki G. Brief ICF Core Sets for the acute hospital. J Rehabil Med 2011;43:123-30.

60. Escorpizo R, Ekholm J, Gmunder HP, Cieza A, Kostanjsek N, Stucki G. Developing a Core Set to describe functioning in vocational rehabilitation using the International Classification of Functioning, Disability and Health (ICF). J Occup Rehabil 2010;20:502–11.

61. Cieza A, Geyh S, Chatterji S, Kostanjsek N, Ustun BT, Stucki G. Identification of candidate categories of the International Classification of Functioning Disability and Health (ICF) for a Generic ICF Core Set based on regression modelling. BMC Med Res Methodol 2006;6:36.

62. Ware JE, Jr., Sherbourne CD. The MOS 36-item short-form health survey (SF-36). I. Conceptual framework and item selection. Med Care 1992;30:473–483.

63. Hudak PL, Amadio PC, Bombardier C. Development of an upper extremity outcome measure: the DASH (disabilities of the arm, shoulder and hand) [corrected]. The Upper Extremity Collaborative Group (UECG). Am J Ind Med 1996;29:602–608.

64. Regensteiner JG, Steiner JF, Panzer RJ, Hiatt WR. Evaluation of walking impairment by questionnaire in patiens with peripheral arterial disease. J Vasc Med Biol 1990;2:142–52.65. Fairbank JC, Pynsent PB. The Oswestry Disability Index. Spine 2000;25:2940–52; discussion 52.

66. Bellamy N, Buchanan WW, Goldsmith CH, Campbell J, Stitt LW. Validation study of WOMAC: a health status instrument for measuring clinically important patient relevant outcomes to antirheumatic drug therapy in patients with osteoarthritis of the hip or knee. J Rheumatol 1988;15:1833–40.

67. Beck AT, Ward CH, Mendelson M, Mock J, Erbaugh J. An inventory for measuring depression. Arch Gen Psychiatry 1961;4:561–71.

68. Folstein MF, Folstein SE, McHugh PR. "Mini-mental state". A practical method for grading the cognitive state of patients for the clinician. J Psychiatr Res 1975;12: 189–98.

69. Mahoney FI, Barthel DW. Functional evaluation: The Barthel Index. Md State Med J 1965;14:61–5.

70. Collen FM, Wade DT, Robb GF, Bradshaw CM. The Rivermead Mobility Index: a further development of the Rivermead Motor Assessment. Int Disabil Stud 1991;13:50–4.

71. Cieza A, Brockow T, Ewert T, Amman E, Kollerits B, Chatterji S, Ustun TB, Stucki G. Linking health-status measurements to the international classification of functioning, disability and health. J Rehabil Med 2002;34:205–10.

72. Cieza A, Geyh S, Chatterji S, Kostanjsek N, Ustun B, Stucki G. ICF linking rules: an update based on lessons learned. J Rehabil Med 2005;37:212–8.

73. Meyer T, Gutenbrunner C, Bickenbach J, Cieza A, Melvin J, Stucki G. Towards a conceptual description of rehabilitation as a health strategy. J Rehabil Med 2011;43:765–9.

74. Muller M, Grill E, Stier-Jarmer M, Strobl R, Gutenbrunner C, Fialka-Moser V, Stucki G. Validation of the comprehensive ICF Core Sets for patients receiving rehabilitation interventions in the acute care setting. J Rehabil Med 2011;43:92–101.

75. Stucki G, Stier-Jarmer M, Grill E, Melvin J. Rationale and principles of early rehabilitation care after an acute injury or illness. Disabil Rehabil 2005;27:353–9.

76. Kirshblum SC, Priebe MM, Ho CH, Scelza WM, Chiodo AE, Wuermser LA. Spinal cord injury medicine. 3. Rehabilitation phase after acute spinal cord injury. Arch Phys Med Rehabil 2007;88:S62–70.

77. Biering-Sorensen F, Scheuringer M, Baumberger M, Charlifue SW, Post MW, Montero F, Kostanjsek N, Stucki G. Developing core sets for persons with spinal cord injuries based on the International Classification of Functioning, Disability and Health as a way to specify functioning. Spinal Cord 2006;44:541–6.

78. Kurtzke JF. Rating neurologic impairment in multiple sclerosis: an expanded disability status scale (EDSS). Neurology 1983;33:1444–52.

79. Antonovsky A. Unraveling the mystery of health: How people manage stress and stay well. San Francisco: Jossey-Bass Publishers; 1987.

80. Antonovsky A. The salutogentic model as a theory to guide health promotion. Health Promot Int 1996;11:8.

81. U.S. Department of Labor EaTA. Dictionary of occupational titles. 4th ed. Washington, DC: U.S. Government Printing Office; 1991.

82. Escorpizo R, Reneman MF, Ekholm J, Fritz J, Krupa T, Marnetoft SU, Maroun CE, Guzman JR, Suzuki Y, Stucki G, Chan CC. A conceptual definition of vocational rehabilitation based on the ICF: building a shared global model. J Occup Rehabil 2011;21:126–33.

83. Jonsdottir J, Rainero G, Racca V, Glassel A, Cieza A. Functioning and disability in persons with low back pain. Disabil Rehabil 2010;32 Suppl 1:S78–84.

84. Grotle M, Brox JI, Vollestad NK. Concurrent comparison of responsiveness in pain and functional status measurements used for patients with low back pain. Spine 2004;29:E492–501.

85. Lauridsen HH, Hartvigsen J, Manniche C, Korsholm L, Grunnet-Nilsson N. Responsiveness and minimal clinically important difference for pain and disability instruments in low back pain patients. BMC musculoskeletal disorders 2006;7:82.

86. Roland M, Morris R. A study of the natural history of back pain. Part I: development of a reliable and sensitive measure of disability in low-back pain. Spine 1983;8:141–144.

87. Waddell G, Newton M, Henderson I, Somerville D, Main CJ. A Fear-Avoidance Beliefs Questionnaire (FABQ) and the role of fear-avoidance beliefs in chronic low back pain and disability. Pain 1993;52:157–168.

88. Yamada KA, Lewthwaite R, Popovich JM, Beneck GJ, Kulig K. The Low Back Activity Confidence Scale (LoBACS): preliminary validity and reliability. Phys Ther 2011;91(11):1592–1603.

89. Deyo RA, Mirza SK, Martin BI. Back pain prevalence and visit rates: estimates from U.S. national surveys, 2002. Spine 2006;31:2724–7.

90. Hashemi L, Webster BS, Clancy EA, Volinn E. Length of disability and cost of workers' compensation low back pain claims. J of Occup Environ Med 1997;39:937–45.

91. Loney PL, Stratford PW. The prevalence of low back pain in adults: a methodological review of the literature. Phys Ther 1999;79:384–96.

92. Walker BF, Muller R, Grant WD. Low back pain in Australian adults: health provider utilization and care seeking. J of Manipulative Physiol Ther 2004;27:327–35.

93. Walker BF, Muller R, Grant WD. Low back pain in Australian adults: prevalence and associated disability. J of Manipulative Physiol Ther 2004;27:238–44.

94. Jette AM, Smith K, Haley SM, Davis KD. Physical therapy episodes of care for patients with low back pain. Phys Ther 1994;74:101–110; discussion 10-5.

95. Hilfiker R, Obrist S, Christen G, Lorenz T, Cieza A. The use of the comprehensive International Classification of Functioning, Disability and Health Core Set for low back pain in clinical practice: a reliability study. Physiother Res Int 2009;14:147–166.

96. Bautz-Holter E, Sveen U, Cieza A, Geyh S, Roe C. Does the International Classification of Functioning, Disability and Health (ICF) core set for low back pain cover the patients' problems? A cross-sectional content-validity study with a Norwegian population. Eur J Phys Rehabil Med 2008;44:387–97.

97. Rundell SD, Davenport TE. Patient education based on principles of cognitive behavioral therapy for a patient with persistent low back pain: a case report. J Orthop Sports Phys Ther 2010;40:494–501.

98. Rundell SD, Davenport TE, Wagner T. Physical therapist management of acute and chronic low back pain using the World Health Organization's International Classification of Functioning, Disability and Health. Phys Ther 2009;89:82–90.

99. Stier-Jarmer M, Cieza A, Borchers M, Stucki G. How to apply the ICF and ICF core sets for low back pain. Clin J Pain 2009;25:29–38.

7 Acknowledgements

Collaborating organizations

World Health Organization (WHO)
International Society of Physical and Rehabilitation Medicine (ISPRM)
World Confederation for Physical Therapy (WCPT)
World Federation of Occupational Therapists (WFOT)
International Society of Prosthetics and Orthotics (ISPO)

Supporting organizations

Abbott Laboratories
Bone and Joint Decade
Center for Obesity, Osteoporosis and Metabolism, Clinic Hirslanden, Switzerland
Deutsche Krebshilfe e.V.
European League against Rheumatism (EULAR)
EU Health Monitor Project Group
French association INTEST-INFO
Gemeinnützige Hertie-Stiftung
German Ministry of Education and Research
German Ministry of Health and Social Security (BMGS)
German Social Accident Insurance (DGUV)
Instituto Carlos III
Institut Guttmann Foundation
German Institution for Statutory Accident Insurance and Prevention in Health and Welfare Services (BGW)
International Labour Organization (ILO)
International Program to develop New Indexes in Crohn's disease (IPNIC)
International Society of Physical and Rehabilitation Medicine (ISPRM)
Ludwig-Maximilians University Munich
LMU innovative project Münchner Zentrum für Gesundheitswissenschaften

Marie Curie Actions of the 6th European Framework Programme MURINET
Nordic Audiological Society (NAS)
OMERACT
Oticon Foundation
Rehaklinik Bellikon (Switzerland)
Schön Clinics (Germany)
SpondyloArthritis international Society (ASAS)
Suva (Swiss Accident Insurance)
Swiss Narcolepsy Society
Swiss Restless Legs Self-Help Group
Swiss Paraplegic Foundation (SPF)
World Confederation for Physical Therapy (WCPT)
World Federation of Occupational Therapists (WFOT)
Zurzach Foundation

Individual participants in the development process of ICF Core Sets

Argentina
Fernando Javier Cáceres
Daniel P. Cardinali
María Josefina Etchevers
Gerardo Rodriguez
Alicia Maria Sambuelli
Carolina Schiappacasse
Gustavo Héctor Vázquez

Armenia
Davit Abrahamyan

Australia
Geoff Abbott
Sharon Barlow
Sian Barry
Lori Beck
Nick Bellamy
Cathy Beveridge
Bernie Bohacik
Carmel Boylan
Douglas Brown
Rhonda Brown
Ann Buchan
Andrea Bucher
Melissa Ceeley
Angela Chu
Andrew Cole
Tanya Cole
Noelene Cooper
Anita Clerke
Craig Crawley
Carol Crocker
Susan Darzins
Leigh Davies
Hugh Dickson
Michael Dillon
Peter Disler
Patricia Dorsett
Diana Dorstyn
Craig Drury
Susan Dunne
Yvonne Fellner
Patricia Fronek
Maria Ftanou
Gary Fulcher
Libby Gibson
Francis Gilfedder
Nicole Grant
Joanne Graves
Stephanie Hammersley
Louise Hatter
Louise Hickson
Phu Hoang
Stephen Hoey
Mark Jones
Amy Keogh
Fary Khan
Friedbert Kohler
Ian Lawrence
Rupert Leong
Wendy Longley
Kay Maddison
Jill Mahar
Laura Martin
Juan-Carlos Martinez

Patricia McAlpine
James McLoughlin
Maria Mercuri
Judith Merritt
Antonina Mikocka-Walus
Libby Morris
Andrew Myers
Robert Newton
Megan Nutt
Jo O'Bree
Lee O´Connell
Tamara Ownsworth
Marilyn Pattison
Garry Pearce
Kiley Pershouse
Loreto Pinnuck
Delaune Pollard
Jennie Ponsford
Emma Power
Patricia Rebello
Joanne Reid
Gail Richmond
Joo Li Robertson
Doug Samuel
Kanit Sananpanich
Sue Shapland
Eva Schonstein
Grahame Simpson
Louise Slater
Caroline Stevens
Margot Strelan
Rodney Sturt
Marilyn Sylvester
Robyn Tate
Anna Tynan
Marina Wallace
Judy Wollin
Linda Worrall
David Worth
Jim Xu

Austria
Edda Amann
Bettina Bauerfeind
Kathrin Ecker
Veronika Fialka-Moser
Susanne Glatzl
Malvina Herceg
Birgit Högl
Karl Knahr
Barbara Kollerits
Martin Krismer
Gabriele Moser
Martin Nuhr
Michael Quittan
Tatjana Paternostro
Christine Prager
Elisabeth Preisinger
Othmar Schuhfried
Attila Simon
Tanja Stamm
Marcus Steinpichler
Johanna Strubreiter
Gerda Vacariu

Bahamas
Ratish Karna

Bangladesh
Ehsunul Ambia
Monjurul Habib
Fazlul Hoque

Barbados
Roslyn Caryl Pearson

Belgium
Raymond Cluydts
Martine de Vos
Gael Delrue
Peter Feys
Denis Franchimont
Frank Goditiabois
Marina Govaerts
Claire Jodogne
Hélène Mathy
Sandra Nuyts
Hilde Verhauwen
Rina Verdoodt
Jan Vermorken
Eric Weerts
Ruth Wittoek

Bolivia
Gonzalo Guillermo Ortuño Ibañez

Botswana
Tlhaloganyo Mbalambi

Brazil
Pola Araujo
Linamara Battistella
Lia Rita Azeredo Bittencourt
Arlete de Camargo
Renata Carvallo
Julia Maria D'Andréa Greve
Julio Maria Fonseca Cheb
Ruy Laurenti
Linda Faye Lehman
Ana Cristina Mancussi e Faro
Carla Gentile Matas
Rose Meire A. Pontes
Marcelo Riberto
Ieda Russo
Eliane Schochat
Alessandra Sousa
Sergio Tufik
Latife Yazigil

Bulgaria
Johanna Jacobson-Petrov

Cambodia
Ka Sunbaunat

Canada
Lindsay Alford
Cate Archibald
Cathy-Lee Benbow
Lise Bouthillier
Denize Brewster-Mellett
Trudy Campbell
Celine Cantin
Kathleen Carr
Frances Chung
Andrea Clark
Susan Conner
Kimberly Cote
Catherine Coulthard
Cathy Croteau
Aileen Davis
Julie Dufresne
Catherine Edgar
Nora Fayed
John Fisk
Susan Forwell
Jean-Pierre Gagné
Isabelle Gagnon
Subhas Ganguli
Michelle Gibbens
Lesley Graff
Anita Gross
Douglas Gross
Linda Gruson
Joan Heard
Janice Hon
Nerissa S Hydal
Branka Jelcic
Mary Beth Jennings
Ania Kania
Michael Kay
Robyn Keon
Marcelo Kremenchutzky
Terry Krupa
Steve Kuyltjes
Andréa Labrecque
Janice Lake
Peter Liao
Caroline Lupien
Rita Mabrucco
Joy MacDermid
Christy Macfie
Amanda Makaryk
Walter Maksymowych
Cathy Mallon
Henry Moller
Mireille Najm
Brenda O'Connor
Jana Popliger-Sinclair
Sophie Provost
Edgar Ramos Vieira
Patricia Rawsthorne
Jennifer Rodgers
Dessa Sadovnick
Fred Saibil
Margaret A. Schneider
Karen Schultz
Mary Sluggett
Michael Sullivan
Joanne Sulman
Andrea Townsend
Judith Thompson
Renata Vaughan
Michelle Wakelin
Elliott Weiss
Shannon Wilkinson

Chile
Pedro Chana
Ricardo Eckart

People's Republic of China
Wei Guorong
Fang Han
Feng Huang
Jianan Li
Patrick Li
Karen Yu Ling Lo-Hui
Jin Bo Tang
Heng Wang
Bing Xia
Xionan Zhou

Colombia
Karim Alvis
Jairo Fernando Gomez
Hernando Laverde-Gutierrez
Julietta Rodriguez-Guzman
Rafaël Valle-Oñate

Croatia
Marko Banic
Vida Demarin

Cuba
Jose A. Cabrera-Gomez
Karina Maria Romero Garcia

Czech Republic
Jana Dusankova
Sona Nevsimalova
Vladimíra Vacková

Denmark
Fin Biering-Sørensen
Tora Dahl
Ulrik Dalgas
Alex de Vries
Anne Dyreborg
Jeanne Hansen

Klaus Krogh
Katja Hagemann Nielsen
Niels Henrik Hjollund
Carina Løvholt Nielsen
Bente Østerberg
Tom Skyhøj Olsen
Björn Sperling
Janni Sleimann Steen

Dominican Republic
Hector Herrand
Marcos Nunez

Egypt
Nirmeen Adel Kishk
Mohamed Farid
Sherif Hamdy
Saher Hashem
Hatem Samir

El Salvador
Carlos Diaz

Estonia
Kombaté Damelan
Heigo Maamägi
Tiina Tammik
Liina Vahter
Inga Zopp

Finland
Leena Alajoki-Nyholm
Hannu Alaranta
Eppu Hokkinen
Tarja Huilla
Sirkka Kolehmainen
Sanna Koskinen
Markku Partinen
Tuula Pirttilä
Eeva-Maija Saaranto
Katarina Stigzelius
Heli Tiainen
Liisa-Maija Verainen
Jos Verbeek
Eeva-Liisa Warinowski

France
Djamel Bensmail
Jean-Frédéric Colombel
Frederic Courtois
Alain Delarque
Liana Euller-Ziegler
Damien Leger
Marc Lémann
Charles Manise
Géraldine Meulin
Alain Muzet
Isabella Nion-Larmurier
Suzanna Ostrec
Benjamin Pariente
Laurent Peyrin-Biroulet
Fabienne Péretz
Aurélie Raust
Florence Salaun
Dan Teculescu

Germany
Ulrike Achleitner
Olaf Adam
Rieke Alten
Christina Andersen
Birgit Basedow-Rajwich
Sebastian Baumann
Sven Becker
Kirsten Becker-Bikowski
Marc Bendach
Alexander Berghaus
Michael Berliner
Stephanie Berno
Antje Beyer
Stephanie Blank
Christine Boldt
Viktor Bonkowski
Tanja Bossmann
Michael Borchers
Jan Brandt
Jürgen Braun
Michaela Braxenthaler
Elke Breitenfeldt
Annette Brink
Thomas Brockow
Petra Brückner
Anne-Katrin Brust
Monika Bullinger
Barbara Busch
Sebastian Canisius
Alarcos Cieza
Michaela Coenen
Paul Cumming
Sergio Crescenti
Trischa Davies-Knorr
Guido Deckstein
Caroline Dereskewitz
Oskar Diener
Andreas Dietz
Karsten Dreinhöfer
Katharina Duddeck
Claudia Dumberger
Andreas Eisenschenk
Jutta Ernst
Thomas Ewert
Hermann Faller
Peter Flachenecker
Karin Forberger
Thomas Franke
Kolja Freier
Wolfgang Fries
Peter Frommelt
Michaela Fuessl
Heinrich Gall

Volkmar Gärtner
Alicia Garza
Catherine Glockner
Eva Grill
Holger Grötzbach
Mathias Grünke
Christoph Gutenbrunner
Andrea Haas
Thomas Harbich
Michael Harder
Ulrich Harreus
Martin Härter
Claudia Hauser
Winfried Häuser
Hilldrun Haibel
Ulrich Hegerl
Rayk Heidbrink
Elke Heinemann
Jörg Heitmann
Thomas Henze
Rudolf Hermes
Ulrich Hildebrant
Andreas Hillert
Christof Hofele
Brigitte Hüllemann
Joseph Ilmberger
Michael Isfort
Wilfried H. Jäckel
Susanne Joisten
Britta Jürgens
Waltraud Kemper
Anne Kenkenberg
Inge Kirchberger
Gernot Klein
Laura Kloc
Stefan Koch
Uwe Koch
Margot Knobel
Hans J. Knorr
Eberhard König
Nicolaus König
Hannelore Kremser-Rüssel
Birgit Kroener-Herwig
Heide Kuhlow
Jochen Kunert
Axel Kunz
Thomas Kurt
Sandra Kus
Sandra Landa
Daniel Langer
Andreas Leib
Klaus Leistner
Werner Liman
Heribert Limm
Elisabeth Linseisen
Joachim Mallinger
Gerson Mast
René Mittrach
Christian Müller
Gertrud Müller
Ines Müller
Martin Müller
Silvia Müller
Ulrike Müller
Andreas Nachtmann
Silvia Neubert
Dennis Nowak
Ralf Nyszkiewicz
Sara Mai Nyguen
Cornelia Oberhauser
Silvia Ostermeier
Antonius Papadimitrakis
Angelika Parentin
Johanna Patika
Andrea Pfingsten
Werner Plinske
Claudia Pott
Anneli Präfke
Gabriele Probst-Eder
Alexander Pröbstl
Philip Quinones
Cornelia Raab
Michael Radoschewski
Alexandra Rauch
Susanne Rauh
Ulrike Ravens-Sieberer
Herman Reigber
Ute Repschläger
Karl-Ludwig Resch
Andreas Römer
Jens Roßmüller
Klaus-Dieter Rudolf
Jörg Ruof
Carla Sabariego
Narine Sahakyan
Kai-Uwe Saum
Hans-Eberhard Schaller
Monika Scheuringer
Stefan Schewe
Hans-Martin Schian
Peter Schöps
Michael Schopen
Maria Schröer
Kerstin Schröter Frey
Gisela Schundau
Wilfried Schupp
Agnes Schuster
Martina Schwab
Sybille Schwarz
Susanne R. Schwarzkopf
Almut Sellschopp
Egbert Seidel
Vanessa Siedek
Not-Rupprecht Siegel
Tanja Sigl
Holger Süß
Annette Stach
Michael Steen
Katharina Stegmüller
Jochen Stelzer

Klaus Stelter
Marita Stier-Jarmer
Irma Stierle
Ralf Strobl
Anette Stolle
Walter Swoboda
Alfred Thilmann
Anne Toenissen
Christine Treitler
Lutz Trowitzsch
Uta Tschiesner
Charlotte Uzarewicz
Sebastian Voigt-Radloff
Sara Wadle
Andreas Wagner
Monika Walchner-Bonjean
Claus Wallesch
Stefan Watzke
Martin Weigl
Frank Werdin
Maryam Wickert
Mathias Wiezoreck
Manfred Wildner
Sabine Wilke
Kai Wingert
Andreas Winkelmann
Markus Wirz
Kathrin Wohlfahrt
Birgit Wolff
Bernt Wünschman
Susanne Zaisserer
Jane Zochling

Greece
Chrysa Chrysovitsanou
Dimitrios Ergeletzis
Patricia Georgakarakou
Zacharoula Mannolidou
Ilias Papathanasiou
Antonios Rombos

Hong Kong
Chetwyn Chan
Sam S Chan
Judith Anne Gould
Wing-yuk Ip
Külli Kaskla
Gladys Leung
Leonard Li
Bradley McPherson
Raymond Tsang
Yun Kwok Wing

Hungary
Geza Balint
Georgina Ilosvai
Lajos Kullmann

Iceland
Elin Ebba Ásmundsdóttir
Valerie Harris
Marga Thome

India
Vineet Ahuja
Pankaj Bajpai
Vijay Batra
Manvir Bhatia
HS Chabra
Abhijit Chandra
Sheela Chitnis
Roopkumar Gursahani
Gita Handa
Suhel Hasan
Sudhir Jha
George Joseph
Moushami Kadkol
Rakesh Kocchar
Abha Kothari
Arun Maiya
Man Mohan Mehndiratta
Sunil Narayan
Bettian Palanisamy
Lekha Pandit
Lilly Farhat Parveen
Vaithiamanithi Perumal
R. Rangasayee
Sumita Rege
Shovan Saha
Preeti Sahota
Alok Sarin
Upinderpal Singh
Ajit Sood
Abhishek Srivastava
Priya Tawde
Lalita Thambi
Sreedhar Thuppal
Noshir Hormusji Wadia
Shiv L. Yadav

Indonesia
Johanes Hardjono

Iran
Noosha Afshinjah
Parisa Ayatollahi
Akram Azad
Mohammad Emami
Malahat Fahimi
Hamid Kamarzarin
Maryam Malekpour
Shahin Merat
Shahriar Nafissi
Mehdi Rassafiani
Noorizadeh Shohreh
Hamd Tavakkoli
Hossein Zabihian

Ireland
Gomathy Ananthan
Yvonne Bailey

Katie Hourigan
Alice McCan
Walter McNicholas
Elaine Neary
Colm Omorain
Julie Regan
John Wells

Israel
Vadim Bluvstein
Eli Carmeli
Yehuda Chowers
Sara Galek
Ofer Keren
Shulamith Kreitler
Ariel Miller
Sandra Neuman
Arie Oksenberg
Haim Ring
Itzhak Siev-Ner
Nachum Soroker
Oded Zmora
Gabi Zeilig
Manuel Zwecker

Italy
Beatrice Aiachini
Ana Álvarez
Paolo Bambrilla
Giacomo Bazzini
Chiara Bertolini
Shaula Bocenti
Oliviero Bruni
Filippo Cavallaro
Marco Cimmino
Gionata Florino
Anna Giardini
Francesca Gimigliano
Alessandro Giustini
Matilde Leonardi
Roberta Litta
Maria Carmen Lonati
Oreste Marrone
Fabiana Marinelli
Gloria Mazzali
Paolo Moretti
Roberta Motta
Giuseppe Palumbo
Piero Porcelli
Caterina Pistarini
Camilla Pisoni
Stefania Pozzi
Silvia Rosso
Marco Songini
Dario Sorrentino
Antonino Spinelli
Paolo Tonin
Rossana Vichi
Mauro Zamboni
Tamara Zamparo

Japan
Toshifumi Hibi
Yuichi Inoue
Shinsuke Katoh
Akira Kimura
Yoshitaka Kinouchi
Takayuki Kondo
Koji Matsuo
Takiji Nagamine
Yuji Naito
Hiroko Ohkawa
Shohei Omokawa
Yoshiko Suzuki
Naoko Tachibana
Masahiko Watanabe
Jun Yaeda
Hiroshi Yamamoto

Jordan
Yousef Ajlouni
Mohamed Elazhary
Imad Gazawi
Waseem Hammoudi
Khaled Jadallah
Ali Otom

Kenya
Julius Nyagah

Kuwait
Abdulla Eyadah
Feroz Khan
Mohammed Nadar

Latvia
Diana Bringina
Zane Liepina
Andrejs Millers

Lebanon
Carole Abboud
Claude Maroun

Lithuania
Alvydas Juocevicius
Andrius Kazlauskas

Malaysia
Tarun Amalnerkar
Victor H. T. Chong
Nazirah Hasnan
Asiah Ibrahim
Chai Hong Lai
Lydia Latif
Irene Looi
Zaliha Omar
Loh Siew Yim

Malta
Bernadette Felice

Mexico
Carmen Alicia Aboytes-Meléndez
Ruben Burgos Vargos
Juan Manuel Guzman
Gerhard Heinze
Carmen Lara
José Antonio Adaya Pérez
Verónica Robles Saucedo
Jesus Yamamoto-Furusho

Mongolia
Ulziibayar Dashdorj
Otgonbayar Luvsannorov

Morocco
Fatima Zohra Ajana
Hamid Ouhabi

Nepal
Prakash Chandra Niraula
Manoj Ranabhat

Netherlands
Frans Albersnagel
Thitus Beentjes
Johannes W.J. Bijlsma
Martin Boers
Annelies Boonen
Alex Burdorf
Marian Curfs
Andrea W. M. Evers
Peter Daansen
Rob de Bie
Jan Geertzen
Mieke Hazes
Yvonne Heerkens
Femke Hoekstra
Sofia Kramer
Tore Kvien
Harry Michon
Marcel Post
Esther Prujis
Ans Rabou
Johannes J. Rasker
Michiel Reneman
Marielle Romberg-Camps
Jan Schouten
Henning Tiemeier
Lucelle A. van de Ven-Stevens
Désirée van der Heijde
Irene E. van der Horst Bruinsma
Sjef van der Linden
Irene van Echteld
Nicole van Erp
Wim van Lankveld
Wijm van Lankveld
Salima van Weelij
Donald L. van der Peet
Gert Walrave
Daniel Wever
Nicolette Wierdsma
Marieke M. Wollaars
Marjolein Zomerdijk

New Zealand
Jennifer Dunn
Janet Freeman
Philippa Gander
Lee Gardiner
Richard Gearry
Paul Hurst
Karen Marshall
Joanne Nunnerley
Michael Schultz
Justine Simmonds
Anne Sinnott
Rachel Stead
Ernest Willoughby

Nigeria
Samuel Ademola
Paschal Ogugua Mogbo
Olulola Oladapo
Fabian Puepet
Solomon Ugoya

Norway
Rune Aarsbog
Søren Brage
Dag Bruusgaard
Nils Fleten
Marit Hjellestad
Erik Bautz-Holter
Lars-Petter Jelsness-Jor
Rikke Helene Moe
Bård Natvig
Simon Øverland
Lillian Reinseth
Cecilie Røe
Tori Smedal
Helene Soberg
Unni Sven
Elisabeth Tvedt

Pakistan
Shaukat Ali
Mahmood Khan
Abdul Malik

Palestine
Rasha Abed
Moussa Abu Mostafa
Yahia Elziq

Panama
María Elena Marquez

Poland
Magdalena Kania
Jarosław Łuczaj
Marek Rogowsky
Joanna Rymaszewska

Portugal
Pedro Cantista
Ricardo Gusmão
Lia Jacobsohn
Luisa Maria Reis Pedro

Qatar
Allen Espelita
Erla Kenway
Monique LeBlanc

Romania
Aurelian Anghelescu
Mihai Berteanu
Alexandru Georgescu
Isabela Lozinca
Mihaela Manescu
Anca Sanda Mihaescu
Luminita Teoaca

Russia
Elena Chashkova
Dmitry Gurevich
Farid Iounoussov
Igor Khalif
Yuri Moustafaev
Irina Osokina
Alexandra Vladimirova

Samoa
Rube P. Une

Saudi Arabia
Ahmed Hassan Al Izzeldin
Imelda Fuentes
Ahmed Hassan
Mariam Misha

Serbia
Petar Bulat
Njegica Jojic

Singapore
Hua Beng Lim
Yeong Ping Peng
Penny Seet
Lay Lay Tan

Slovenia
Dusan Baraga
Helena Burger
Darja Fiser
Alenka Höfferle-Felc
Jelka Jansa
Alenka Kobal
Crt Marincek
Maja Ogrin
Mojca Prusnik
Andreja Švajger
Lea Zver

South Africa
Alison Bentley
Lila Bruk
Tania Buys
Robert Campbell
Gillian Coetsee
Johan Fagan
Andrew Girdwood
Theresa Gouws
Rushda Hendricks
Tabitha Hume
Wendy Lewis
Hermann Liebenberg
Ayesha Mahomed
Girish Mody
Lee Randall
Carla Janse van Rensburg
Rene Smalberger
Michael Solomons
De Wet Swanepoel
Dorothy van der Spuy
Lizelle van der Vyver
Corrianne van Velze
Hester Margaretha Vermaa

South Korea
Yoo Soon Bang
Chang Soo Eun
Hyun Sik Gong
Eunsil Kim
Young Ho Kim
In Sik Lee
Nam Jong Paik
Keunchil Park
Soo-Kyung Park
Hwang Seongsoo

Spain
Celia Anaya
Carolina C Ávila
José Luis Ayuso-Mateos
Marta Gallego Barrero
Helena Bascuñana
Jesús Benito
Miguel Benito
Montserrat Bernabeu
Mariá Cabello
Eva Cobos
Salvadora Delgado
Consuelo de Dios
Juan Lopez Diaz
Eloy Espin

Elena Ezquiaga
Alberto Garcia
Carlos Gonzales
Marta Renom Guiteras
Matilde Hernandez
Antonio Torrejon Herrera
Sara Laxe
Itziar Leal
Mariana López
Raquel Lopez
Anabel Martínez-Arán
José Manuel Montes
Blanca Mellor
Eloy Nin
Enrique Noé
Ingrid Ordàs
Ricardo Pagan
Victor Pérez
Ana de Pobes
Jesús Rivera
Pablo Rodríguez
Susana Rodriguez
Teresa Roig
Marcos Riíos Lago
Rocio Sánchez-Carrión
José Sanchez Moreno
Estibaliz Terradillos
Josep M. Tormos
Carla Torrent
Jesús Valle
Antonio Veronese
Joan Vidal
Eduard Vieta

Sri Lanka
Kemal Deen
Janaka de Silva
Udaya Ranawaka

Sweden
Kristina Akesson
Beatrix Alguren
Catharina Broberg
Jan-Erik Broman
Sonja Calais van Stokkom
Maria Carlström
Berth Danermark
Lotta Dellve
Elin Ekbladh
Jan Ekholm
Kristina Schüldt Ekholm
Ulrika Englund
Ingemar Engström
Sarah Granberg
Gunnar Grimby
Margareta Gustafsson
Lena Haglund
Lars Hansson
Lena Hartelius
Björn Jakobsson
Pia Malcus Johnsson
Ann-Katrin Karlsson
Eva Månsson Lexell
Stefan Lohmander
Sven-Uno Marnetoft
Claes Möller
Roland Morgell
Anna Nilsdotter
Eva Roos
Gunnel Sandqvist
Bengt Sjölund
Henrik Stjernman
Jan-Peter Strömgren
Katharina Sunnerhagen
Frank Wollheim

Switzerland
Andrea Albiez
Bernd Anderseck
Felix Angst
Deniz Aras
Giuseppina Areniello
Andre Äschlimann
Cornelia Bachofner
Carolina Ballert
Claudo Bassetti
Christian Baumann
Michael Baumberger
Gabriel Benz
Stéphanie Bessard
Jerome Bickenbach
Ursula Biland-Thommen
Heike Bischoff
Eveline Bodmer
Cristina Bostan
Roberto Brioschi
Ulrich Bürgi
Mirjam Brach
Nathalie Braun
Teresa Brinkel
Sandra Brueren
Maurizio Calcagni
Somnath Chatterji
Philippe Cottagnoud
Neisa Cuonz
Olivier Deriaz
Nandini Devi
Alissa Dress
Gerold Ebenbichler
Brigitte Egli
Karl Emmenegger
Nicole Emmenegger
Peter Erhart
Reuben Escorpizo
Margrit Fäßler
Yvonne Fernandez
Klaus Fetscher
Rene Fiechter
Monika Finger

Daniela Fuchs
Nina Geiser
Carl Gennheimer
Christian Geyh
Szilvia Geyh
Kurt Gfeller
Edith Gitermann
Andrea Glässel
Hans Peter Gmünder
Matthias Gugger
Elly Hengeveld
Ulrike Hoffmann-Richter
Lisa Holper
Inge Eriks-Hoogland
Fritz Horber
Erika Huber
Jacqueline Huber
Chantal Huguenot
Hans Jörg Huwiler
Giuseppina Jacovo
Robert Jakob
Beatrice Jansen
Bruno Keel
Jürg Kesselring
Ramin Khatami
Andreas Klipstein
Christina Knellwolf
Otto Knüsel
Barbara Köhler
Jan Kool
Nenad Kostanjsek
Kaba Dalla Lana
Thomas Langenegger
Franco Lanfranchi
Veronika Lay
Helga Lechner
Hansjörg Lüthi
Miriam Lückenkemper
Christian A. Ludwig
Kurt Luyckx
Johannes Mathis
Christine Meier
Philippe Merz
Franz Michel
Federico Montero
Rachel Müller
Barbara Murray
Karin Niedermann
Arto Nirkko
Diana Nix
Rahel Oertli
Peter Oesch
Iris-Katharina Penner
Claudio Peter
Lucien Portenier
Natascha Potoczna
Pavel Ptyushkin
Barbara Rau
Geoffrey Reed
Jan Reinhardt
Klaus Resch
Stefan Ritler
Gilles Rivier
Gerhard Rogler
Corinne Roth
Markus Roth
Philipp Rückheim
Wolfgang Schmitt
Hans Schwarz
Urban Schwegler
Wolfgang Segerer
Melissa Selb
Jana Skoblikova
Anna Sonderegger
Stefan Staubli
Frank Staudenmann
Monika Stocker
Thomas Stoll
Katherine Strasky
Armin Stucki
Gerold Stucki
Urban Studer
Nicole Suter
Maurizio Trippolini
T. Bedirhan Üstün
Claude Vaney
Inge-Marie Velstra
Martin Verra
Beat Villiger
Annamarie Vogt
Per von Groote
Bernd Wagner
Martina Walti
Ulrich Weber
Yvonne Wechsler
Andrea Weise
Christian Wenk
Niklas Wiegand
Gabriela Winkler
Balz Winteler
Beat Wunderlin
Gaby Wyttenbach
Heidi Zimmermann-Heinrich
Genevieve Zurbriggen

Syria

Ahmad Khalifa

Tanzania

Dominick Michael Mshanga

Taiwan

Yin-Chih Fu
Kwan-Hwa Lin
Shwu-fen Wang
Yen-Ho Wang
Hui-Ching Wu
Mingyi Wu

Thailand
Tuenchai Attawong
Preecha Chalidapong
K Y Rebecca Chan
Piyapat Dajpratham
Morakot Intasarn
Supalak Khemthong
Naiphinich Kotchabhakdi
Apichana Kovindha
Jirachart Kraisarin
Somporn Onlaor
Naraporn Prayoonwiwat
Somporn Pan Sungkarat
Puntarica Suwanprathes
Piya Trevittaya
Sirikan Yamada

Togo
Djamiou Oumorgou
Kimberly Obst

Trinidad
Jacqueline Rouse

Tunesia
Catherine Dziri

Turkey
Hatice Acar
Emel Aydın
Okan Caliyurt
Aysegul Colakoglu
Hüseyin Engin
Ilke Keser
Ali Kitis
Deran Oskay
Gunes Yavuzer

United Kingdom (including England, Northern Ireland, Scotland and Wales)
Mark Agius
Michael Barnes
Julie Barlow
June Beharry
Neil Betteridge
Tom Burns
Paula Cowan
Paul Dieppe
Wagih El-Masry
Jenny Freeman
Lynda Gettings
Jane Giles
Clare Ginders
David Good
Felix Gradinger
Karen Holbrook
Jain Holmes
Ian Hindmarch
Gerry Humphris
Nicola Hunter
Alan Izat
Jane Johnson
Marie Johnston
Paul Kennedy
Jill Lloyd
Fiona Lobban
Miranda Lomer
Stanton Newman
Christopher Nutting
Robin Pickard
Jenny Preston
Miles Rinaldi
Kerry Robinson
Simon Rogers
Anita Rose
Justine Schneider
Nick Slevin
Toni Stamp
Millicent Stone
James Stubbs
Fiona Sudgen-Best
Catherine Sykes
Deborah Symmons
Anitra Thomas
Dot Tussler
Sheena Visram
Derrik Wade
Anthony Ward
David Warwick
Anthony Woolf

United States of America
Rhonda Abbott
Renato Alarcon
David Arciniegas
Peter Arnett
Richard Atkinson
Anthony Ayag
David Beck
Morris Bell
Keith Bengtson
Francois Bethoux
Gary Bond
James Bowen
Brent Braveman
Jan Burnes
Lester Butt
Michele Capella McDonnall
J. Catesby Ware
Susan W. Charlifue
Ian Chen
Toni Chiara
Kevin Chung
Evan Cohen
Janice Colwell
Noreen Comeau

Adele Crudden
Antonio Culebras
Terry DiLorenzo
Charles E. Drebing
Sharon Dudley-Brown
George Ehrlich
Bruce E. Ellerin
Alberto Esquenazi
William A. Faubion
Michael Feuerstein
Alessandro Fichera
Marcia Finlayson
Julie Fritz
Gerry Funk
Russell Gelfman
Barbara Giesser
Christian Guilleminault
Andrew Haig
Manny Halpern
Elizabeth M. Hannold
Karen Hanson
Jutta Hinrichs
Mark Johnston
Debra B. Homa
Cinda Hugos
Brian Hutchinson
Karen Jacobs
Rosalind Kalb
Leonard Kamen
Sunanda V. Kane
Jeffrey Katz
Anthony J. Kerrigan
Robert Steven Kistenberg
Nicholas La Rocca
Edward Levine
Edward Loftus
Paul Lysaker
Kay Maddison
James F. Malec
Ruth Ann Marrie
David J. Martin
Deborah McCloskey
Alan McGuire
John Melvin
Deborah Miller
Linda Moore
Douglas Moul
Ari Mwachofi
Dot Nary
Margareta Nordin
Brittany Norton
Darrell S. Pardi
John Pemberton
Walter Penk
Inder Perkash
Scott Plevy
Jamie L. Pomeranz
Monika Reimitz
Scott Richards
David Ring
Gianna Rodriguez
Tammy Roehrs
Rick Roessler
Ann E. Rogers
Bonnie Rogers
Phyllis Ross
Thomas Roth
Ernest M. Roy
Michelle Rubin
William J. Sandborn
Steven Schwid
Jackie See
Joseph Sellin
Patricia Soliz
Matthew Sorenson
Joseph F. Stano
Alexa Stuifbergen
Matthew Sutliff
Jeffery Sybert
Pat Tracy
William J. Tremaine
David Vandergoot
John Wadsworth
Nicolas Walsh
Rick Wickstrom
Roberta Winter
Heather Wishart
Bruce Wolff
John Whyte
Edward Yelin
David A. York
Bevan Yueh
Nathan Zasler

Uruguay
Beatriz Lade

Vietnam
Cam Hong Linh
Ha Van Than
Dinh Quang Thanh

Zambia
Margaret M. Mweshi

Zimbabwe
James January
Megan Mutepfa

8 Key Terms

9 Contents of Enclosed CD

1. ICF Core Sets

(a) Acute Healthcare Context (Brief and Comprehensive)
- Acute Arthritis
- Cardiopulmonary Conditions
- Musculoskeletal Condition
- Neurological Conditions

(b) Post-Acute Healthcare Context (Brief and Comprehensive)
- Cardiopulmonary Conditions
- Geriatric Patients
- Musculoskeletal Conditions
- Neurological Conditions
- Spinal Cord Injury

(c) Long-Term Healthcare Context (Brief and Comprehensive)
- Ankylosing Spondylitis
- Bipolar Disorders
- Breast Cancer
- Chronic Ischaemic Heart Disease
- Chronic Widespread Pain
- Depression
- Diabetes Mellitus
- Hand Conditions
- Head and Neck Cancer
- Inflammatory Bowel Diseases
- Low Back Pain
- Multiple Sclerosis
- Obesity
- Obstructive Pulmonary Diseases
- Osteoarthritis
- Osteoporosis
- Rheumatoid Arthritis
- Sleep
- Spinal Cord Injury
- Stroke
- Traumatic Brain Injury
- Vocational Rehabilitation

(d) Generic Set

2. The Documentation Forms for All ICF Core Sets

(a) Acute Healthcare Context (Brief and Comprehensive)

- Acute Arthritis
- Cardiopulmonary Conditions
- Musculoskeletal Condition
- Neurological Conditions

(b) Post-Acute Healthcare Context (Brief and Comprehensive)

- Cardiopulmonary Conditions
- Geriatric Patients
- Musculoskeletal Conditions
- Neurological Conditions
- Spinal Cord Injury

(c) Long-Term Healthcare Context (Brief and Comprehensive)

- Ankylosing Spondylitis
- Bipolar Disorders
- Breast Cancer
- Chronic Ischaemic Heart Disease
- Chronic Widespread Pain
- Depression
- Diabetes Mellitus
- Hand Conditions
- Head and Neck Cancer
- Inflammatory Bowel Diseases
- Low Back Pain
- Multiple Sclerosis
- Obesity
- Obstructive Pulmonary Diseases
- Osteoarthritis
- Osteoporosis
- Rheumatoid Arthritis
- Sleep
- Spinal Cord Injury
- Stroke
- Traumatic Brain Injury
- Vocational Rehabilitation

(d) Generic Set

3. Use Cases

(a) Use Case 1: Applying the ICF Core Set for Patients with Musculoskeletal Conditions for Acute Care
(b) Use Case 2. Applying the Comprehensive ICF Core Set for Spinal Cord Injury for Post-Acute Care
(c) Use Case 3: Applying the ICF Core Set for Multiple Sclerosis
(d) Use Case 4: Applying the ICF Core Set for Vocational Rehabilitation
(e) Use Case 5: Applying the ICF Core Set for Low Back Pain